Caring for Your Voice

Teachers and Coaches

E. L. (Betty) Donaldson, Editor

Detselig Enterprises Ltd.

Calgary, Alberta, Canada

© 1995 E. Lisbeth Donaldson

Canadian Cataloguing in Publication Data

Main entry under title:

Caring for your voice

Includes bibliographical references.

ISBN 1-55059-119-3

1. Voice – Care and hygiene.   2. Communication in education.   I. Donaldson, E. Lisbeth (Ethel Lisbeth).

RF510.C37 1995   612.7'8'024372   C95-910581-6

Detselig Enterprises Ltd.

210-1220 Kensington Rd. N.W.

Calgary, Alberta, Canada

T2N 3P5

Cover Design by Bill Matheson.

Printed in Canada   SAN 115-0324

Table of Contents

Detselig Enterprises Ltd. appreciates the financial assistance received for its 1995 publishing program from the Department of Canadian Heritage and the Alberta Foundation for the Arts, a beneficiary of the Lottery fund of the Government of Alberta.

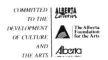

Preface

To listen to the teacher's voice in the classroom is to listen to the heartbeat of the educational system. Communication between teacher and student reflects the value that society places upon encouraging youthful talent, transmitting the cultural heritage and developing societal mores. Nevertheless, like many people, teachers may not like the sound of their own voice. It may sound more authoritarian than authoritative. Another group of professionals, coaches, have an image of themselves as being almost indestructibly strong, and they expect their voices to represent this image. Both teachers and coaches use and misuse their voices frequently because they haven't learned about caring for their voices.

Thus, the book title became *Caring for <u>Your</u> Voice.* As teachers and coaches think about "the" voice they use when working in professional environments, they've acquired "a" voice with regard to the unique demands associated with their professional responsibilities. At the core, it is a recognition of the personal, and individual, in each voice.

Purpose of the Book

The purpose of this book is to encourage teachers and coaches to take better care of their voices. By caring for their voices, they take care of themselves and communicate better with other people. Teachers and coaches are two groups of "professional voice users" whose needs have not been well addressed. Thus, problems emerge that affect personal health and erode professional practice. For those who do evolve good vocal habits, the rewards are many. They feel better generally, they speak fluently, and they are effective motivators. A voice is as individual as a fingerprint or a footprint: it represents a unique aspect of the person. Adopting any suggestion from the following chapters will be taking one step toward expressing such individuality.

Other audiences for this book are students enrolled in professional schools. Future teachers, coaches and speech pathologists need to understand how to care for the voice. If during their early careers, they develop good vocal habits, they will avoid many of the problems mentioned here. In addition, they will be better communicators.

Need for the Book

This book evolved from surprise and concern. Surprised that teachers and coaches were so uninformed about a major occupational hazard, I began to talk about voice fatigue and pathology with other professionals who had similar interests. Although absenteeism rates in schools because of laryngitis and associated vocal problems are very high, little has been written about care of the voice for teachers and coaches. In dry climates especially, vocal problems are the most frequent reasons for missing work or changing professional practice. Speech pathologists know that during the Spring season the percentages of teachers and coaches among their patient loads increase.

For professionals who depend upon their voice to make their livelihood, the thought of being speechless is frightening. Nevertheless, many think that a summer or seasonal break will rest their voice – and it does. Thus, teachers and coaches may ignore warning signs and symptoms for many years. Finally, some have treatment or surgery. The suggestions in this book are aimed at reducing or avoiding such health problems among teachers and coaches.

There is a further concern. People who do not have good voices are difficult to listen to. Therefore, the teacher's voice is a classroom tool that, like any tool, must be honed and maintained. Furthermore, as with any personal characteristic, it may be developed to its maximum. Teachers and coaches know very well they are role models for their students and athletes. They constantly use their voices to encourage development of talent. In this book teachers and coaches are urged to develop their individual voices for their own benefit as well as for those they mentor. It simply is good professional practice.

Overview of the Contents

The book has five chapters, each authored by professionals with an interest in voice, but who write from differing perspectives. The chapters provide a continuum of insights ranging from interviews with teachers and coaches regarding their professional practice, suggestions for professional development, reducing vocal problems and pathology, and an alternative approach in voice therapy. In each chapter, insights based upon professional expertise are offered, and each concludes with suggestions for pragmatic readers. Chapter One is focused upon teachers: their professional development regarding voice, classroom management and school-based environments. Suggestions from teachers who have been working to reduce vocal problems make an important contribution because pre-service students and colleagues will listen to these voices. Chapter Two provides rare insights about how professional coaches use and misuse their voices. Essentially, Don McGavern issues a wake-up call. Chapter Three is packed with exercises for those who want to develop their voice. Readers may benefit whether or not they have an opportunity to attend the workshops offered by Janine Pearson and Kelly McEvenue at Stratford Festival. Chapter Four is based on years of working with patients who have developed vocal problems. Speech pathologists Alanna McDonough and Elizabeth Hunt understand very well the resistance that teachers and coaches have toward changing lifestyle habits and the motivations for doing so. In Chapter Five, Marcia Epstein describes some of the changes that result when clients make connections between previous life experiences and voice problems. Chapter Six will be "written" by those who utilize suggestions from the previous authors.

Scope of the Book

This book contributes little to the extensive literature on public speaking and speech arts, but it does draw from expertise in these areas. Professionals in the performing arts, people who give speeches and those travelling conference circuits already know of the many books they might consult. Thus, while the scope of this book is limited to an audience that may not realize the need for professional development of the voice, perhaps alert browsers might refer friends and acquaintances who would benefit from a read. It's even possible that alert browsers might find some suggestions useful when caring for their voice.

Acknowledgements

As editor, I acknowledge the commitment of the authors and publisher. From the first meeting with Ted Giles of Detselig Enterprises Ltd. no one missed a step in the dance toward completion of the project. Along the way, we all coped with full-time work schedules and personal responsibilities. Janine Pearson and Kelly McEvenue had previously worked together at Stratford Festival but during most of the time they authored their chapter, Janine was in Quebec and Kelly in Ontario. Alanna McDonough and Elizabeth Hunt have never met; as professional speech pathologists, Alanna is employed in Alberta and Elizabeth has a practice in Ontario. During the writing of their chapter, each had a daughter, born five weeks apart in Spring, 1995. Welcome, Isabelle and Courtney: we look forward to hearing more of your voices. Don McGavern, Marcia Epstein and I are grateful to the professionals who shared their stories with us; some names appear in our respective chapters while others are anonymous. To Linda Berry, publisher's editor, all authors express gratitude for patience and particularism. Thank you also to the support staff and institutions that provided environments which nurtured the project: the University of Calgary, the National Theatre School and Stratford Festival, the Foothills Hospital and the Voice Centre in Toronto.

E. L. (Betty) Donaldson
Calgary, Alberta, 1995

CHAPTER 1
Reflecting Upon the Teacher's Voice
E. L. (Betty) Donaldson

Ask for a definition of "the teacher's voice" and professionals wince. Most teachers immediately think of a strident, authoritarian image they prefer to avoid, but remember times when it's necessary to issue a command. Some dislike the sound of their own voices when listening to a taped version because they don't think it's "them." A few have never thought much about how they speak; their concern is with the lesson plan.

I began reflecting about the teacher's voice while observing pre-service teachers present in communication classes and in practicum situations. Their voices often sounded thin as if they were frightened. Some spoke too quickly or too much. Others had voices so faint they couldn't be heard although a few boomers could make anyone freeze. High pitched voices appeared whiny while low voices snarled. These people had invested years in earning degrees to qualify as professional teachers, but they didn't know much about using their voices as a professional tool. Not surprisingly, classroom management was a problem. Then I learned that many of my graduate students and friends in the teaching field had serious vocal problems, and some required surgery. Yet, all were familiar with the concept of voice and dedicated to developing their students' voices, especially in writing assignments. Why were professional teachers so intellectually committed to the psychological voice and so naïve about the physical voice? How might the psychological and the physical voices be connected? Perhaps the gap could be bridged.

This chapter contains a brief review of relevant literature about "voice," reminds teachers that they are professional voice users and summarizes some teacher voices of experience. It concludes with a few strategies that might be used to reduce vocal problems and to develop a better classroom teacher voice. However, the chapter is really an invitation for further reflection.

Types of Teacher Voices

Recent literature about voice has assisted students and teachers to discover their "voice," by which is meant facilitating individual growth and validating the authenticity of personal experience. When the individual story is also the history of an alternative perspective, such as pedagogical narratives or the women's movement, the statement has political as well as personal connotations. However, while this trend encourages development of the psychological voice, connections with the physical voice are not always recognized.

Teachers interested in facilitating the development of a personal voice often are involved with various writing activities, such as the Calgary Writing Project, which is a network of teacher-consultants who work locally, nationally and internationally to encourage staff development through collegial exchanges. Another trend is the concept of personal narratives as the process by which curriculum is understood, shaped and delivered (Connelly & Clandinin, 1988). Both approaches acknowledge the primacy of an inner voice that develops as a result of life experience and conscious reflective practice. It opposes and contrasts a stance based upon objectified, standardized knowledge that is the external framework by which students and teachers are most often evaluated. The clash between the two perspectives stimulates much of the most dynamic thought and current research about educational reform.

During the 1970s interdisciplinary research between the fields of composition and cognitive psychology stimulated a paradigm shift among those who teach writing. Students were encouraged to move from a writer-based orientation to reader-based prose by using various problem-solving strategies. This approach is now challenged by social constructionist research which emphasizes the importance of context in understanding events, developing "meaning" and influencing interpretation (Buss, 1993). Also, occasionally a dissenting voice appears such as Donald Stewart's argument for an "authentic" voice: "I suspect that one of the late twentieth century's reasons for distancing itself from writing with an intensely personal voice is not only our era's worship of the scientific and technological fact and the mania we have for presenting it uncontaminated, but an even deeper and unexpressed need to avoid confronting the essential shallowness of our spiritual lives. . . . we make a serious pedagogical mistake when we do not acknowledge [that any good writer has a single identifiable voice running beneath all his or her work] and encourage our students to develop their own voices as far as they are capable of doing so." (Stewart, 1992, p. 288).

The women's movement has generated considerable, and influential, literature about interrelationships between self, voice, mind and psychological development. Carol Gilligan (1982) notes that women make ethical decisions based upon relationships more than do men, thus they speak in a different voice. Mary Belenky identifies different types of subjective and procedural knowledge that result in "voices" which need to be integrated (Belenky, Clinchy, Goldberger & Tarule, 1986). Deborah Tannen (1990) argues that women's and men's voices represent cross-cultural dynamics which create misunderstanding and conflict as well as intimacy and insight. Finally, it seems appropriate to acknowledge Nel Noddings' insight that, ethically, teaching moments are "caring occasions" (Noddings, 1988). When women care for their own voices, their "teacher voice" more fluently reflects their caring for the children who are their students. The many efforts of women not to be silenced in their personal and professional lives and to express a voice representative of their gendered life experience is transforming society.

What's interesting in this brief review of literature about voice is the realization, despite the profound impact these perspectives have had upon pedagogy, and upon personal and professional development, how little attention has been directed toward the speaking voice. The psychological voice, as articulated in writing, cannot automatically be assumed as identical to the spoken word, either in process or in content. For many reasons, people talk differently from how they write. The process varies even when the topic is constant. Similarly, while the speaking voice undoubtedly reflects psychological status, especially emotions, it would be simplistic to assume one "voice" exactly mirrors others. Nevertheless, connections between these voices continue to intrigue writers, dramatists, psychologists and educators.

There is a need for thoughtful dialogue about how to understand our respective voices as our society enters a phase in which local and regional attachments to community weaken while commitment to the global village grows. Families struggle to share time, meals and thoughts, but children and parents spend hours at a computer playing electronic games or sending e-mail. People telephone, but speak to a tape recorder or growl about voice mail messages. Distance education, home schooling and charter schools permit access to knowledge, but the limited range of interpersonal contacts may restrict acquired wisdom. Interactive technology encourages machine interface, but allows people to avoid daily interpersonal communication. In a planet that is home to more people than ever before, more are isolates within their own communities. Thus, the teacher's voice in the classroom becomes the oral voice of the culture. It represents an ancient tradition.

Professional Voice Users

The tradition of public speaking evolves from ancient cultures dependent upon oral historians. People in those societies listened well, had good memories and revered good storytellers. When the best way of learning something rests upon the fragility of the spoken word, those who speak well become the shamans, the elders, of the tribe. During the five centuries of the printed word, communication became more segregated into personal and public spheres. Within the public sphere, lectures, entertainment and persuasive sales pitches became dominant modes of presenting information. Thus, public speech became more impersonal, frequently involving one person speaking to an audience comprised of people who weren't known to the presenter (Cooper, 1994). A classroom has elements of both oral and print traditions and will undoubtedly be changed once again by the electronic revolution.

In the classroom, teachers are the shamans, the elders, of our tribe. It's the professional responsibility of teachers to induct young people into full citizenship; furthermore, most teachers think they have a responsibility to cultivate a love of learning that results in lifelong enrichment. Children need to be informed, entertained and persuaded. Experienced teachers know how to shape intellectual material, to plan a variety of pedagogical strategies and to use a sense of humor. But they rarely think of *how* they will speak about their topic.

Common to both oral societies and public print traditions are an understanding of the body as a speech instrument, an appreciation of the range of emotions in the audience and an ability to organize the intellectual message (Safire, 1992). They also love the sound of words. But, all too often, teachers do not listen to the *sound* of their words. In addition, most teachers plan lessons well; good teachers also understand emotions, but only a few teachers prepare their bodies for daily speech activities. While many teachers appreciate fitness as a personal goal, they don't always connect that value to classroom communication. Furthermore, although general fitness raises energy levels, it doesn't always result in better vocal habits.

Not participating in any physical activity, drinking lots of coffee as a tonic and ignoring the aging process are behaviors that put teachers' voices at risk. Gradually, they realize they suffer more colds or flu, dread the classroom schedule and are more frequently absent from extracurricular activities, meetings and school. Some visit the doctor, complaining of sore throats, raspy voices and vocal fatigue. A few develop polyps or nodules on their vocal folds that must be surgically removed.

While some teachers have vocal problems during the Fall, they assume they'll be "fine" after the start-up period has conditioned them to school demands once again. Then, in the spring, they're tired and presume that a rest during the summer will be sufficient. Over a period of years, this cycle may intensify, with recovery periods becoming more brief and less effective. Speech pathologists know the percentage of teachers among their clientèle increases in spring as the school year ends. In some instances, the percentage increases from a third to two-thirds of their practice; in drier climates the numbers are higher. Apparently, the most frequent reasons for teacher absenteeism are vocal problems such as hoarseness, sore throat and voice loss. Motivation for changing one's lifestyle – or teaching style – increases with a diagnosis of a pathological problem, but it is possible for many teachers to persist with borderline habits for a long time, partly because holidays provide rest and relaxation periods that allow them to retain a marginal level for years. It's not unlike the gradual fadeout cycle of a dropout student: the pattern is obvious, effective intervention is more difficult.

Unlike teachers, performing arts professionals, such as singers, dancers and actors understand the demands upon their bodies. They know they must train for performances that demand peak action at the outer ranges of physical limitations. Singers practise to extend their vocal range, to hold notes "effortlessly," and to project melodic vowel sounds. Dancers stretch their bodies from neck to ankle and practise movements expressing joy, sadness and surprise. Actors establish a physical presence that is not always vocal, using space, timing and projection. For each of these professions, daily warm-ups and a clear understanding of body dynamics are part of the vocation. Their vocations depend upon their voice. In fact, the word "vocation" derives from the same root word as "vocal" and "vocabulary." "Professional" contains the word "profess," which evolved from "confess": an oral public statement about one's views. Given this definition, teachers are unquestionably professionals in a demanding vocation!

In studies of occupational success, speech abilities are always highly ranked, and teachers often are remembered more for the personality they project than for the subjects they teach. Often this assessment of personality rests upon student perceptions about what type of person the teacher is as reflected by what's heard in her or his voice. Is this person warm or cold, interesting or boring, caring or bossy? Sometimes, students are attracted to or repelled from a subject or course content according to their response to a teacher's style. "I love chemistry because Mrs Worthwhile was so enthusiastic, so interesting. She likes showing me how to do it." How did the student know about this teacher's commitment? By hearing these qualities in her voice.

A teacher may begin to assess "speech personality" by asking "why is 'good speech' important in 'good teaching'?" (Fessenden, Johnson, Larson & Good, 1968, p. 19). Self-reflective evaluation could be initiated by answering questions such as these examples:

- Do I succeed in putting people at ease by the way I speak?
- Is my speech pleasant, easy to listen to? Or is it harsh, strident and unpleasant?
- Is my speech faulty in any respect? Do I have a pronounced regional accent? Do I articulate clearly? Are the syllables distorted? (Fessenden et al., 1968, p. 311)

Perhaps the following headings would be a valuable prompt for journal writing. Note how closely they relate to good classroom management:

Voice quality	**Correct language usage**
Social effectiveness	**Range of Inflection**
Oral reading ability	**Enunciation**
Skill in story telling	**Skill in conversation**
Questioning skills	**Listening skills**

Teachers continually discuss strategies that develop good practice; however, they don't talk as often about voices that "inspire." Few would deny the psychological connection between the "breath of life" or the inner "voice" that informs the "good life." Similarly, "to be spirited," or "filled with spirit" means to be animated, to have breath, energy, a presence. (Although, in Spring, some teachers wish some students had less!) Murray Schafer, a noted Canadian composer, argues that life is a multimedia experience and that obtaining *A Sound Education* (1992), develops auditory awareness to help us understand our environment, improves our listening skills and increases our delight in being alive. Therefore, when thinking about the professional voice of teachers, it's wise to remember also that silence is part of the communication cycle and a component of good speech.

Effective Teacher Strategies

While teachers share problems common to all voice users, they also need to articulate solutions appropriate for educators. Once pathology is diagnosed, speech therapists have an array of exercises to alleviate symptoms. However, prevention not only reduces discomfort and disease, it is the best model for developing a voice that becomes a more fluent teaching tool, reflecting an extensive teaching repertoire and a learning stance toward life itself.

At the beginning of an In-Service course on caring for the voice, I asked a group of experienced teachers to complete this statement: *When I think about my voice I am mainly concerned about* . . . They wrote about the need for:

- developing variety in tone in order to use it well for class management;

- having control when anxious or under stress;

- projecting so that the tone and expressiveness are not overpowering to those nearby but audible at a distance;

- discovering ways of preserving the voice on a daily basis;

- knowing whether my education is reflected in my voice and my choice of words;

- avoiding loss of my voice or experiencing strep throat this year;

- not doing irreparable damage to my voice, vocal cords or developing cancer of the throat through the abuse that I know my vocal cords take;

- finding ways that I can use my voice more effectively to motivate, stimulate and share my enthusiasm with the students;

- preserving the speaking timbre, the attractive quality of my voice.

- knowing what I really sound like.

Several weeks later, they offered solutions: ideas they'd applied during their practice and in their daily lives after reflective self-assessment. Their solutions may be grouped into three categories: changing personal lifestyle habits, addressing specific points of tension in the body and refining new classroom management strategies.

One new graduate, who had taken several public speaking courses, continued to feel vulnerable. She decided she "pulled back" when speaking, drawing in energy rather than sending it out. Connected to this problem was a tendency to preface comments with "Just a quick question" or to append them with "I think." She made the psychological connection to a lack of confidence, but she also reduced her caffeine intake and increased physical activities such as jogging. Then she deliberately selected times to speak out when she felt challenged but not threatened. Gradually, she realized she could express emotions through her voice, "reminding myself it is my right to be heard."

An experienced teacher realized that she was most likely to have headaches on Wednesdays and Thursdays so she developed a deep relaxation routine to use at bedtime. Integrating relaxation and appropriate breathing into a team-teaching situation was more difficult, however both teachers developed a signal system for the grade one/two class. Keeping their voices calm, using hand signals, they said "And stop," emphasizing the vowel "A." They discovered that by the time they'd finished "stop," the students were silent and listening. After saying "Thank you" they moved on to the next activity.

A male administrator, who for several years had had canker infections that resulted in serious sore throats, was responsible for lunch supervision in a gym of 450 children. He initiated a daily routine that began with a gentle massage of the facial muscles, especially the jaw area. After some tongue and jaw stretch exercises, he drove to work using a tape he'd created to guide him through vocalization and breathing exercises. He quickly revised this routine because initially he was overenthusiastic and attempted too much while the vocal muscles were still flaccid. Several weeks later, he arrived at school feeling good and ready to start the day, knowing he had built up a weak area of his body to the point where it met daily demands more easily.

Four of the teachers in the course focused specifically upon bodily tensions they knew they had. "Besides being an over-worked, underpaid, stressed out teacher, I knew that there might be other reasons for my rapid speaking rate," wrote one grade 10 teacher. "Having 39 students who, at times, ap-peared rather listless, restless, inattentive and not overly excited about how to protect Canada's sovereignty certainly contributed to an increased speaking rate." After analyzing times when "life in the classroom was calm," she began visualizing being centred during moments when she felt rushed. Making a deliberate attempt to drop the shoulders, relax the spine and inobtrusively wiggle the jaw, she also stood quietly at the front of the room, noting how it drew student attention. She visualized her voice filling the room with clear, unhurried directions, and practised key instructions using varying inflections. She also asked students to project when speaking. "Using these simple techniques has brought me fame and fortune, students clamouring to be let into class and then sitting on the edge of their seats hanging on to my every word. Well, not exactly. It has, though, made me more con-scious of how the voice can create an atmosphere that is a positive influence on learning." Another teacher knew she watched the rearview mirror when driving rather than doing an over the shoulder check. She worked on head and shoulder relaxation, combined with breathing and postural alignment when she was in bed at night. Then she applied her relaxation strategies in the classroom, waiting quietly until students were aware she was not talking. She was surprised to discover how quickly they came to attention while at the same time she gave her voice a rest and avoided the anger cycle that contrib-uted to a stiff, tense neck and shoulder pattern.

Another teacher developed a set of jaw and tongue exercises that combined breathing patterns. These included chewing motions (as if eating crackers) that lead to voiced words such as "candy chunks, cherries and peaches." After several yawn sighs, she'd add vowel sounds. Using hiss movements with her lips, she practised inhaling and exhaling. As a result, she thought her voice became more musical – a quality she wasn't taking for granted.

A high school math teacher used a tape recorder in her class to analyze her "voice personality." Friends and husband confirmed the nasal quality that she had been dismayed to hear. To help correct this problem, she practised vocalizing sentences that had nasal sounds, plus ones with no nasal sounds, holding her nose while she did so. Gradually, the nasal vibrations became different when the sentences changed. In front of a mirror, she practised mobilizing her uvula (soft palate), until she could hear the difference. Using the tape recorder to check periodic progress, she concluded, "It's like I have discovered another voice – it seems richer and more pleasant to listen to. . . . There is no room greater than the room for improvement."

Four teachers focused upon classroom management strategies. One junior high teacher enlisted her students' support because she knew they didn't like "subs." Explaining that she'd be absent less frequently if they cooperated, she timed the length of the class response after she'd asked students to listen. From the instant she said, "I'd like your attention, please," to total class silence never took less than 53 seconds. "Psychological time, as every teacher will attest, is very different from Swiss watch time and I use the extra minute to breathe." She also used hand signals such as making a circle in the air to indicate the "wrap-up" minute had commenced. Flicking lights, "hands in the air: mouths closed" routines are common nonverbal signals, but her new insight was that they also are methods that allow her to take care of herself. "The students know when a classroom is too noisy. And most of them don't like it. So, in some ways they become my voice (when they warn each other). I can save mine for teaching or explaining, or reminding, or congratulating. The warning part of classrooms always was the part I liked the least anyway."

A music teacher used wooden sticks to attract student attention. She also split the choir into two groups. Also, she practised waiting for silence, working on dynamic body alignment while doing so. Finally, she began doing the exercises with the children, reasoning, "If it is good for me it should be good for them." A teacher who had a girl student who tended to scream in class involved the entire class in making decisions about changed vocal behavior. The children decided to carry water bottles, they agreed upon a hand signal that signified silence, and they spoke with voices that carried only a brief distance when working in groups: their "15 cm voice." Within several weeks, she noted that there were fewer requests for washroom breaks or drink breaks between classes, screaming rarely occurred, and everyone, including herself, spoke more quietly. A elementary physical education specialist experimented with nonverbal strategies, such as students saying "last girl or last boy" out of the change room, while she stood holding a small basket, silently smiling and making eye contact as students deposited jewellery and watches. When the children were to group for instructions, she quietly counted down 5-4-3-2-1, watching with incredulous eyes as they moved quickly into a circle around her. In the classroom, instruction periods began with the lights off; turning the switch on meant silence, the class had begun.

One Teacher's Story

The teachers who worked so diligently to make lifestyle changes, reduce bodily tensions or revise classroom management strategies were motivated to avoid discomfort and disease as well as to improve the learning environment in their classrooms. They are more fortunate than a teacher who was forced to make these changes after surgery for nodules on her vocal folds. Fifteen years later, Brenda Wallace, seconded to the University of Calgary as a university associate responsible for practica supervision, thinks she's a better professional, with a more extensive range of teaching repertoires, but she'll never forget her eight days of silence after surgery.

Brenda grew up in a farming community in Saskatchewan. As the eldest girl in the neighborhood, she organized games for the little boys; as a talented musician, she began teaching piano lessons when in grade seven. After graduating from university, she taught physical education and music in Saskatoon to elementary and junior high school students. When she moved to Alberta and joined the Calgary Board of Education, she continued to specialize in these subjects. She used her voice extensively and enthusiastically. As a coach, she'd do intramural pep talks. On the playing fields she "could stop a student dead in his tracks 100 yards away." As a music teacher she lead singing groups on television and in musicals. Ten years later, having had two children, she had good general health, but was missing school 25 days a year because of chronic bronchitis. In those days, secondhand smoke in the staff room was "lethal" so she avoided it, but frequently she suffered throat infections. Finally a specialist diagnosed "singer's throat," nodules on the vocal cords. "I was banging my vocal cords together, creating blisters that became infected. When any germs came around me, I became ill." During the Winter of 1980, she had surgery and people came to her house to watch her "not talk." She was known for her "teacher talk," competing with students for air time.

People had complimented her on the distinctive quality of her voice, "its huskiness." When she began speech therapy, she realized she had "to say good bye to a whole lot of things I'd done previously." As she retrained her voice in the therapist's office, reading aloud in higher pitch, trying to avoid stimulating a flashing red light, Brenda acknowledged that the commanding, deep voice she'd developed to sustain the phys. ed. image was gone. She could no longer work in cold gyms, switching between indoor and outdoor activities with ease. Nor could she continue to lead boys' choirs in raucous songs.

The "good news" is that "I haven't missed school due to illness for years." Determined to break the cycle of sore throat, low energy and illness that had plagued her for a decade, Brenda gave up coaching outdoor activities, began teaching social studies and explored new classroom management strategies. Brenda continues to play the piano, so "I'm part of the music," but she doesn't sing any more. Eventually, she began to coach basketball because it is an indoor activity. However, her enthusiasm is expressed through nonverbal signals such as stamping her feet, clapping or raising her hands, and smiling with lots of direct eye contact. She's learned the value of vocal naps.

In the classroom, she signals rather than raising her voice. When junior high students ask, "Ms. Wallace, how come you never get mad?" she laughs. "I get mad, but I get quiet when I get mad. My students know that when I'm silent, that's the time to pay quick attention." Brenda thinks the tone she establishes in the classroom is very important to discipline and to teaching. She likes to start the class "at a nice place," so she avoids scolding and repetitious reminders. It's a part of her pedagogical philosophy that the classroom is a community of learners. Thus, she models enthusiasm, cooperation and curiosity about learning social studies. And, she has "pre-thought" process as well as content carefully for the school year, for the week and for daily activities.

She knows that in September or after a holiday, she is more likely to have a sore throat. So, she uses "my little tricks" to make her voice last. At the beginning of the year, she clearly explains her expectations to the children: they're told to watch for hand signals; they're warned to be quiet when she asks for silence. While Brenda likes cooperative learning activities, she doesn't do group work at the beginning of the term.

Brenda Wallace has become an expert in using space, time and nonverbal communication to save her voice. Desk patterns are changed at least three times a week. A table is placed behind the desks to avoid the typical adolescent drift toward the back of the room away from the teacher space. She uses rows only during tests. Usually student desks are organized into circles, u-shapes or three semi-circles staggered around a video or activity centre. A favorite arrangement is the sunshine pattern: she sits on a stool with the students arrayed in front of her. When she does move into group work, the students change a room in under 5 seconds. "They love it. There's a great crash of moving desks." However, before the students move into a new pattern, she carefully explains the procedure, making certain that all are in a position to watch her face. When she is certain that everyone understands the directions, then she uses a stop watch.

During basketball season, the day begins at 7 a.m. because of coaching responsibilities. At 8 o'clock, classes begin. Each of the five classes has 28-33 grade nine students; the daily agenda has been written on the board so students do not need to ask what is next. During lunch hour and recess, there are various supervisory activities while preparation time is used for one on one tutoring, marking or lesson planning. In addition, Brenda's teenage daughter is active in a number of sports activities so she attends events, providing parental support. As well, Brenda and her husband share a love of sailing. Her schedule is busy.

It's a relief that, for the past 7 or 8 years, staff rooms are no longer so smoky because her throat "hurts almost im-mediately." When in such a situation, she moves into her high pitch voice, maintaining the same volume and rate as she normally uses. However, she tries to avoid coughing, prefer-ring instead to swallow. When her throat feels dry, she drinks a lot of water and chews gum, permitting her students to do the same providing they respect the community environment. When the classroom is dry, she uses a tea kettle to increase humidity.

Brenda thinks it's important to distinguish between under-ground noise and student noise. Underground noise is the sound of the classroom: outside distractions, fans, intercom announcements, feet scraping the floor. Student noise results from talk and chatter. Some underground noises can be reduced. For example a carpet helps maintain a quieter environment. Class begins with the lights off; when they are turned on, it's time to start working. By contrast, student noise can be controlled. When working in groups, the conver-sational level is acceptably high. But students also work alone in timed seven minute modules during which there is silence, and she makes a point of not interrupting them. "Lost time" in the classroom is the bane of every teacher, but Brenda has timed these periods and discovered they're frequently less than one minute. She accepts this loss as inevitable, balanc-ing it with "savings" in patience and voice care. Silence is valued with the knowledge that a voice that punctuates silence is a more effective teaching tool than one which is constantly running on with few interruptions.

It's important to be fresh for the last class of the day because "it's not fair to them if I'm tired." She has several focal points in the classroom, moving frequently between them while maintaining a conversational tone and proximity to all students. One focal point is a lectern; another is a desk; a third is the blackboard. A comfortable chair, reading light and tv are at the back of the room, providing a restful place. A favorite prop is a high stool because it allows her to see all the faces around her while stretching her torso so she breathes easily. At another time she may be sitting at a table, with students looking over her shoulder watching her work at a project.

Brenda is a slender, active person with a mobile, bright face who likes to greet her students at the classroom door. She has penetrating eye communication which never wavers during one on one conversation. Her hand signals are crisp and unambiguous. "I'm out and about in my classroom. And, I'm a better teacher than when I was using my voice all of the time. I've got more variety." Smiling with satisfaction, she concludes: "There's nothing more enjoyable than a room of grade niners totally silent, focused upon a task. A teacher who speaks with a soft voice can create a soft atmosphere, one that makes learning pleasurable. I can't imagine what it would be like not to use my voice to express my emotions and my enthusiasm." Brenda Wallace's teacher voice is not loud and strident, but it is authoritative, knowledgeable, filled with affection for her students and pride in her profession. As a university associate, she models this type of teacher voice as one that new teachers could cultivate. She's learned to make connections between her psychological and physical voices for the benefit of her students, her teaching style and her personal goals. While her style is unique, a reflection of her personality, her strategies could be adapted by any teacher interested in caring for his or her voice.

Concluding Suggestions

Teachers interested in cultivating a speaking voice, one that reduces pathology and enhances the classroom learning environment, need to begin by reflecting upon their environment, their bodies and their speaking voices.

School buildings tend to lack humidity and harbor germs. The numbers of people using these facilities generate a public exchange of diseases as well as ideas. Therefore, an analysis of the daily schedule develops a focus on what might be the most effective strategies for a particular environment. If the classroom is an echo chamber, as many gyms are, nonverbal communication and quiet voices make the atmosphere more tolerable. Thirty sets of eyes silently waiting for another group to join them is a powerful influence. In a room where sound is muffled, handouts and posters might be appropriate supplements to brief presentations. The library is a quiet place; hallways and playgrounds are not. When a classroom is more like a library, one can take a vocal nap; when the classroom is noisy, one need not shout. Flicking lights, standing quietly, writing a note on the blackboard, using a soft bell are good alternatives to making more noise than 30 children. Some teachers like to use whistles; others consider them barbaric. Pre-planning works. Thinking about the weekly schedule during Fall and Spring semesters helps establish a personal routine appropriate for the season. Individual regimes vary as do peak demands. The car is a good place in which to warm up the voice, even if the neighboring drivers might notice a teacher making faces while the traffic light is red.

Probably gender makes a difference. In my work, male teachers and administrators have been more reluctant to discuss their vocal problems, offering reasons both personal and professional. Their feelings of vulnerability are obvious; their desire to work out their difficulty privately is apparent. By contrast, women teachers immediately begin to problem solve, to discuss concerns and to share insights. There seems to be little gendered difference with regard to how these teachers conduct professional responsibilities; nonetheless, female and male voices differ in tone, pitch, volume and resonance. Unquestionably, the sound of the teacher's voice reflects gender, but the impact upon students may be more educational mythology than pedagogical fact.

Variety is one key to successful classroom management. Understanding space, time and voice intersections helps to establish an environment in which students thrive. Rotating between activities such as small group exercises, silent reading or individual oral work rests the teacher's voice while developing essential communication skills. Using students to quieten each other frees the teacher to observe covert problems. Trusting silence – and timing the length of periods that seem long – helps develop the range of vocal pacing during a period and can make a few words more effective than many.

Students should be taught to savor the sound of words, especially ones such as "dawn, luminous, murmuring, tranquil and golden," some of the most beautiful words in the English language when spoken aloud. Contrast them with "mugged, screech, gripe and jerk." Imagine how much students would learn if they appreciated the sound, as well as the origin, of five to ten key words in any subject. Not only would they have a knowledge of basic concepts they should remember, they probably would integrate a mnemonic aid that permits them to recall a constellation of ideas and applications.

Teachers with reduced levels of energy feel tension in the bodily systems that produce voice. They sound low as well as feel low. They may breathe poorly and literally run out of "gas" (i.e., oxygen). It's worthwhile remembering the old words "hale" and "hearty" when "in/haling" or "ex/haling." Quite literally, we are more hale if we breathe appropriately because the lungs and heart filter and pump oxygen throughout the body to generate energy. Tension, however, reduces energy, and habitual tension in a particular area of the body reduces the flow of freshly oxygenated blood to that area. Our physiological health influences our psychological health and vice versa. Knowing how to relax – generally and specifically – releases energy that can be redirected. Relaxation doesn't necessarily lead to deep sleep; it can reduce stress in challenging situations. Teachers cannot control everything that occurs in a classroom, but they do have choices about their types of response. Like most skill development, however, practise is necessary (Hiebert, 1993).

The voice may be a teaching "tool" or a pedagogical "instrument;" nevertheless, it is a unique sound generated by an individual body. Vocal warm-up exercises could be rotated accordingly. However, voice exercises are most effective when the entire body is "warmed up" or, conversely, relaxed. Knowing where habitual patterns of tension are located within the body creates awareness. Because teachers prepare so well intellectually for their work, a frequent pattern is head and shoulder immobility. It's difficult to speak well through a neck that is tight, a jaw that doesn't move, and a tongue that is stiff. Sometimes teachers lock their knees to maintain a stance or dig in their heels. The bodies of most people eventually reflect occupational stresses and strains. Teaches need not be stiff marionettes and most aren't. Everyone, however, benefits from knowing where personal tension is habitually stored in the body and how that pattern might be caused by occupational stress.

Facial muscles need to be mobile "masks." A television commercial claims it takes 43 muscles to frown and only 17 to smile: why work harder than necessary! Maintaining sufficient breath is essential; while not a difficult skill to learn, it may be hard to apply in situations that evoke tension. When in a busy classroom, just learning to breathe from the centre of the body while not lifting the shoulders would immeasurably benefit most professional educators. Using knees and ankles as mobile springs that contribute to nonverbal communication consumes less energy than stiff legs and contributes to a sense of being ready to deliver a worthwhile message.

The importance of nonverbal communication as an adjunct to a good teaching voice has scarcely been explored. However, the value of organizing physical facilities for maximum pedagogical benefit is recognized. Lights, carpets, desk arrangements, board and wall messages can be used to enhance vocal messages, to complement them, or to reduce teacher talk. Hand signals, facial expressions, body stance and feet movements illustrate and amplify verbal communication. All teachers know how effective this level of message can be, but few have thought about how their teaching style might be adapted if speech patterns were integrated with hand, body and foot movements. In addition, spatial patterns could be reviewed: activity centres, small group dynamics and student leadership skill development distribute learning responsibilities, but don't exhaust the teaching voice.

Videos, film and audiotapes are commonplace classroom tools, but the effects of computers and voice mail have not been studied much. Certainly, in a multimedia environment, students and teachers will be much more aurally literate, as well as being oral and visual sophisticates. Without a doubt, in an electronic classroom, what constitutes "voice" will be different from a print-based schoolroom. "The sound of silence" will change as asynchronous time messages left on e-mail and telephones indicate someone is listening but not at the moment, while real time messages become more brief as the result of reduced response times conditioned by electronic beeps and individualized schedules. Given this scenario, the teacher's voice will change. Perhaps there will be less demand for sustained teaching in physical plants that are not conducive to prolonged vocal demands; perhaps daily classroom periods will be longer or shorter. Even the length and time of the school year may be altered. Whatever the changes, teaching will remain a category of professional voice usage, and teachers will need to care for their voices.

Many teachers will not begin to practise vocal care until they have acquired problems. However, prevention is the best "model" because an extended teaching style evolves as the voice becomes more fluent. Teachers with diagnosed vocal problems will receive advice from physicians, speech therapists or other health care professionals about how best to deal with the specific syndrome. For general problems regarding volume, range, pitch and tone, the following suggestions may be useful. Volume, the loudness or softness relative to a situation, depends upon breath. To have volume sufficient for a 25 foot range, posture that helps the diaphragm push sufficient air through the larynx is necessary. This posture must be maintained during movement as well as during a static position. Rate, the speed with which words are spoken, should vary according to the emotional content of a lesson: even a science lesson can have suspense. Long presentations may be punctuated with vocal naps, brief silences or questions. Pitch is the range of "musical notes sung" during ordinary speech. Most people never extend that range, attempting to express all feelings within a narrow band that approximates a monotone or jumping quickly to an extremely loud command from a low-voiced explanation. Making humming sounds from within the mouth helps extend the normal range beyond one octave (eight notes). Tone is the resonance or vibration that adds quality to the voice. Vowels "spoken" from cavities in the head, face, nose, throat, and chest sound different to both speaker and listener. The result is a rich voice, well worth listening to: a vocalized rainbow of sound.

Preventing problems from occurring is the best way to develop a vocal range that is a career asset. After thinking about some aspects that might be changed, it's useful to ask other people, trusted colleagues, friends or family, for feedback in situations as differing as the classroom, the hallway or the field trip. Most people don't like the sound of their own voice, and they never hear themselves as others do. It's possible to recognize echoes between the physical and psychological but remember that, just as the mind is not identical to the brain, the voice is but an indication of the self and the soul. Listening to an audio or video tape of one's voice is risky unless self-assessment skills are quite balanced. Tapes are, nonetheless, invaluable reinforcers because they record improvement, providing rewarding comparisons.

"There is no index of character as sure as the voice," said British Prime Minister Benjamin Disraeli. Like most good quotations, while not necessarily a true statement, the nugget of truth reminds us of a profound value. Teachers voice the ideals of society. When these voices have strength and good pacing, reflecting range and resonance, students are more willing to accept the responsibilities of citizenship by learning curricula and are more challenged to develop their talents by participating in assignments. The voice of the teacher reflects the range of values in our culture: psychological and physical, intellectual and spiritual. When the teacher's voice expresses such qualities, students learn well.

References

Belenky, M., Clinchy, B., Goldberger, N. & Tarule, J. *Women's Ways of Knowing*. New York: Basic Books, Harper Collins Publishers, 1986.

Buss, H. *Mapping Our Selves*. Montreal & Kingston: McGill-Queens University Press, 1993.

Cooper, B. *Speak with Power*. Calgary: Pow'r Publications, 1995.

Connelly, M. & Clandinin, J. *Teachers as Curriculum Planners*. Toronto: OISE Press, 1988.

Fessenden, S., Johnson, R., Larson, P. & Good, K. *Speech for the Creative Teacher*. Iowa: W.M.C. Brown Company Publishers, 1968.

Gilligan, C. *In a Different Voice*. MA: Harvard University Press, 1982.

Hiebert, B. *Learn to Relax. A Step-by-Step Guide*. Calgary: Lugus Books, 1993.

Noddings, N. An Ethic of Caring and its Implications for Instructional Arrangements. *American Journal of Education, 96*:2, 1988, pp. 215-230.

Safire, W. *Lend Me Your Ears, Great Speeches in History*. New York: W.W. Norton & Company, 1992.

Schafer, M. *A Sound Education*. Ontario: Arcana Editions, 1992

Stewart, D. Cognitive Psychologists, Social Constructionists, and Three Nineteenth Century Advocates of Authentic Voice, *Journal of Advanced Composition, 12*:2, pp. 279-90, Fall, 1992.

Tannen, D. *You Just Don't Understand*. New York: William Morrow & Co. Inc., 1990.

E. L. (BETTY) DONALDSON, Ph.D., is Associate Professor in the Faculty of Education, University of Calgary. Coordinator of the pre-service communication courses, she teaches graduate courses in communication, women in education and administration. In her first career, she was a physiotherapist, specializing in neurophysiological development and psychosomatic disorders. As an educator, she has taught and administrated in various school boards, colleges, technical institutes and universities. She has taught canoeing and is past-president of the Canadian Recreational Canoeing Association and of the British Columbia Recreational Canoeing Association. For a number of years, she has also been involved in theatre as a producer, playwright and as a volunteer.

Chapter 2
Reflecting Upon the Coaching Voice
Don McGavern

As a sport coach, I am amazed how silent the profession has been regarding the care of development of the "coaching voice." A year ago, after being associated with coaching and the teaching of physical education classes for over thirty years, I was severely stricken with a form of "chronic vocal disorder" (CVD). Up to that moment I had used my voice "liberally" in a variety of decibels for the purposes of motivating, encouraging and providing feedback to athletes and students in environments not conducive to normal vocal ranges, i.e. gymnasiums, outside fields and swimming pools.

While developing chronic hoarseness and raspiness last year, I was not remotely knowledgeable or concerned about any short and long term implications associated with the possible misuse of the vocal system. My intent is to share, not only my story, but some experiences of others in the field of physical education who have experienced similar voice afflictions or limitations during their career.

This chapter is a reflection upon the uses and misuses of the coaching voice in athletic and physical education environments. The focus is not to present a program of therapy, as I am not a trained specialist in this field. What follows are three case studies of "career coaches," in addition to responses from six teachers of physical education from Calgary. The Physical Education teachers have been identified using their first names only, with their permission. All who were interviewed developed symptoms or problems related to CVD, i.e., hoarseness, loss of vocal power, soreness of the throat area and even loss of the voice. However, the ways they communicated to their athletes or students, in conjunction with the unique demands associated with teaching "of the physical" in training and competing environments were very similar. To those who participated, my deepest thanks for their time and help in allowing me tell their stories so that others might benefit.

The Case of Don McGavern
Diving Coach and Teacher of Aquatics
Physical Education

Background

Don McGavern is the Manager of Aquatics and a member of the Teaching Faculty for the Faculty of Kinesiology at the University of Calgary. He has been associated with the Faculty since 1984. McGavern earned his Master of Science degree in Physical Education at the University of Oregon. While at the University of Oregon, he was the varsity intercollegiate diving coach and an assistant professor in the School of Health, Physical Education and Recreation specializing in the instruction of aquatic courses. He moved to Canada in 1973 to become the National Technical Director for the Canadian Amateur Diving Association where he helped develop the national learn-to-dive program in addition to initiating the national coaching certification program for the sport. In 1979 he moved to Edmonton, Alberta, to resume active coaching in the sport of diving at the club level. His athletes competed at the provincial, national and international levels. He was a national junior and senior team coach for Team Canada. His last major international diving coaching assignment was with Team Canada in 1986 at the World Aquatic Championships in Madrid, Spain. In 1987, he retired from active coaching in the sport of diving. Currently he is a volunteer community basketball coach, an active course instructor in the Canadian National Coaching Certification Program and operates his own consulting business as a public presenter, conducting workshops and seminars to business and sport groups on motivation and enhanced personal performance.

The Story

In January, 1994, I had completed a particularly exhausting week of teaching and coaching activities, including: fifteen aquatic classes in a variety of disciplines, all offered in a fifty metre complex; two evening basketball practices for eleven- and twelve-year-old boys; two evening community classes presenting coaching theory; a weekend coaching assignment at a basketball game; and a weekend public speaking presentation. Similar past teaching and coaching experiences usually resulted in a hoarse voice on the following Monday and Tuesday. However, by Wednesday, my voice would return to normal, or at least what I construed to be normal.

My life has always been full of active "vocal communications" operating at a variety of decibels to pass encouragement, enthusiasm, motivation and critical teaching points on to my athletes. As a teacher and coach in the outdoor environment of track and field and the indoor environment of the aquatics field, I have always spoken to my athletes and students in a loud and forced manner, partly due to what was deemed to be a normal "coaching voice" for those environments, in addition to matching a normal part of my coaching and teaching personality. Over the years I experienced hoarseness and voice fatigue on several occasions, especially at the start of the training and competition season or during a week of competition. With a week's rest, my voice usually recovered.

However in this 1994 instance of vocal overuse and fatigue, the hoarseness did not disappear after a week's rest. In fact the voice condition did not improve during the next four weeks. My voice had been reduced to a "gravelly whisper." Thinking I had developed a form of laryngitis, I went to see my family physician, assuming that some form of antibiotic and resting of the voice would be the treatment. After a preliminary examination, my physician suggested that although there was no sign of laryngitis, the throat was definitely inflamed, strained and injured. He referred me to a throat specialist.

When one is referred to a "specialist" in medicine, there is always the possibility that the ailment is much more serious than a sore throat and strain. I remember vividly exercising my imagination that day while driving to the specialist. Negative visualizations of nodules on the vocal cords, possible medical alternatives such as an operation, and a lifetime continuation of hoarseness and limited vocal power "danced in my head." In addition to those negative thoughts, I kept reviewing all previous moments in my life when similar diffi-culties had occurred in order to determine what might have caused such discomforts. I did not have a history of the more common conditions that one would normally associate with a sore throat, such as long term smoking, allergies or chronic laryngitis problems.

Upon arriving at the specialist's office, I was not encouraged environmentally to abandon my negative thoughts. While waiting in the general patient area, I scanned some of the notices on the bulletin boards. Included were notices for a variety of weekly and monthly meetings for those who had lost their voice. In addition, there were advertisements for special devices that could replicate normal voice sounds. After scanning such notices, I immediately started talking just a little bit louder so that my preliminary examination would be deemed only a "sore throat."

If you've never been to a throat specialist to have your throat examined, then the thrill and fun of having a probe light extended down your throat is awaiting you. If I had known that good vocal training and preventive care might have prevented this experience, I know that I would have been much more diligent about it in my younger years. Even after "freezing" the throat area, no experience yet equalled having the throat specialist place the inspecting tube, with a light on the end, deeply into my throat to view the vocal cords. Keeping my mind calm to avoid a regurgitation reaction reinforced my coaching beliefs that there really is a need for mental training in maximizing physical performance. In this instance, I am sorry to report that I did not compete well.

After the examination, the throat specialist said that my vocal cords had indeed become enlarged and inflamed; in addition, he noticed growth of nodules caused by overuse. He gave me medication to reduce the inflammation and recom-mended reducing vocal activities where overuse was likely. He also indicated that if there was no improvement before the second examination, in about one month, he would recom-mend a speech therapist.

By the time of the second examination, about seventy five per cent of my voice power had returned, so I was feeling a lot more optimistic about "surviving." My assumption was that it had just been overuse and that the quality, tone and power would return in time, as in the past. I was so optimistic that I had even been practicing for the second inspection of the throat area. The second insertion was a small improvement in that I experienced less physical discomfort; however, the specialist said that there was still some evidence of nodules. He thought it would be best for me to meet with a speech and language pathologist and referred me to the Foothills Hospital in Calgary.

I am not sure if other coaches are like me in the area of seeking personal medical help, but I for one am quite reluctant to do so. Pride and "being tough" always seemed to make me avoid seeking medical counsel unless I severely ill and physically disabled. On the opposite side of the coin, I am very quick to see that the medical needs of my athletes are met.

When I knew that I was being referred to a "therapist," I felt instant relief that my vocal dilemma did not require surgery. Because I felt that major treatment had been averted, my mindset prior to the first meeting with the speech therapist was somewhat casual and indifferent. In fact, I can remember thinking that the examination would probably be cursory, somewhat simple in analysis and I would be given a clean bill of health with a recommendation for a quick and speedy return to my professional environment.

My therapist was Ms. Alanna McDonough, a certified language and speech pathologist in charge of voice pathology at the Foothills Hospital in Calgary. She first reviewed my particular situation. Then she presented information about the structure of the voice, the vocal cords and how sound was transmitted. She also used "buzz words," related to the use of voice, that were foreign to me, even though I had used my voice extensively in coaching, teaching and public speaking presentations. She talked about "placement," "voice or pitch level," "breathing" and "body posture for effective vocal control." She had me read several passages which would reflect the qualities expected of a "healthy voice."

After the readings she suggested that I did have some voice problems. If they were not corrected by changing certain vocal patterns, long term problems might surface. Her initial recommendations including "listening to" and "feeling" the various sounds of the voice as they were emitted in relation to the exhalation of air. She showed me that I was holding my breath, especially on louder words, phrases or sentences. I was using the nasal or front portions of my voice, which restricted air flow across the vocal cords, producing strain. As I ran out of air, a "gravelly" tone resulted. We practiced "placing" the voice and changing the "pitch level" using different sounds or words that commonly reflected this nasal response.

Finally, she recommended that I start "watering the throat," called "hydration." This regime included drinking six to ten glasses of water throughout the day, but especially during times of "heavy voice use." Since I was a "sports person," using a water bottle was not inconvenient or unfamiliar. Along with the hydration, she suggested I work on my breathing related to several vocal sounds and make a conscious effort to listen to the area from which the sound was emitting.

Needless to say, after that preliminary one-hour vocal session, I was astounded at my naïveté regarding proper voice sounds and care. It was as if I had just been awakened to some very basic truths, known by everyone but me. Had I known, I believe I could have prevented many past misuse situations from occurring earlier in my career. That initial meeting with Alanna was the beginning of what is known in the self-development field as a "life shaping event."

Alanna provided handouts detailing the use of the voice, in addition to several exercises. For the first two weeks I concentrated on digesting and applying the new information to its fullest. I practiced every day, sometimes three to four times a day. I attempted to reduce the number of times that I was forcing my voice. I also practiced "talking out loud" with various work sounds and sentences Alanna had given me. I used every opportunity available. Sometimes I practiced in the car while traveling to and from work. While physically exercising, I practiced during rest periods, taking several full and deep breaths to emphasize proper exhalation techniques. I even practiced taping my voice on a portable tape recorder while walking our family dog, listening to the playback in an effort to produce more proper sounds.

On my second visit I had improved in certain areas, but I returned home to continue practicing my breathing and reading exercises. This time I was to experiment with various voice levels, starting with a whisper and moving to an above-normal voice as used in coaching situations. It was during this second period that I started to miss practice sessions. As with dieters or those who begin exercising or even those who want to find time for anything dealing with self-improvement or change, unless there is a strong conscious internal drive to attain a certain level of proficiency, daily efforts will not be consistent. Unfortunately, I felt that I had now accomplished the basic concepts of correct voice training. Believing that I had, I thought further daily voice training efforts and repetitions could be reduced and diminished.

On my third visit, Alanna, like any "experienced coach," spotted the ineptness of my practice and training, noting that certain vocal patterns were returning. She said that to guarantee a positive vocal future, I had to be the catalyst, meaning I had to be a coach as well as a trainee. The program of pitch, placement and controlled breathing must become a life experience, not one quick set of exercises. If not, I would continue to experience more moments of CVD afflictions, eventually leading to major problems. These problems of vocal misuse could amplify with age. In conclusion, Alanna indicated that since I had recovered approximately ninety percent of what is considered a normal speaking voice, continued visits would not be necessary unless there was a relapse. Compared to most cases that she dealt with, I would be considered "very normal." However, I should not take her diagnosis as an indication that "practising" could stop.

I have not been back to Alanna for over a year. The information with which she provided me will now always be a core part of my daily life activities and events. Whether I continue to practice all of the exercises as much as I should remains to be seen. However, I have already noticed some significant changes to previously "normal behavior patterns" which have resulted in decreased throat strain. Some of the new "life habits" include:

1. hydrating on a regular basis throughout the day with **water**, especially during moments of high vocal intensity, such as when I am orally presenting or during

competitions in which I am coaching. Lukewarm water "feels" better than ice water, especially when I have to sustain the talking mode.

2. using a greater variety of hand signals and similar non-verbal communication techniques. These "visual cues" are shared with the athletes and students at the beginning of the season, class or whenever the time is appropriate. After communicating and sharing my vocal problems with my athletes and students, they help me keep "vocal cues" in perspective by reminding me whenever I "lose it."

3. setting some time aside at the beginning of any major presentation or time period in which my voice will be extensively used, to do a lot of visual imagery and breathing exercises for a "vocal warm-up."

4. not clearing my throat when there seems to be congestion. I try first to breath in from the nose and then the mouth.

5. practising a variety of the self-help drills that Alanna gave me. For example:
   a. "relaxing the voice" through sounds that open the throat on inhalation (deep full breaths), and then relax the vocal cords on exhalation by slowly sighing "ahhs" and "uuus" until all of the air is expired.
   b. practicing with words which bring the voice up, such as "hello," "really" and "ready."
   c. practicing phrases that use a "humming" or vibration of the vocal cords in conjunction with breathing. Some of my favorites are: "many, many, many," "man in the moon" and "night time moon."
   d. exercising slowly and then trying for the same sound when the pace is changed to a faster tempo.
   e. producing complicated sounds with which the inexperienced voice can have difficulty, especially in clarity. Some of my favorites from Alanna's sessions include: "raspberry patch," "peach tree plaza" and "wreath of roses." I also use tongue twisters, both slow and fast in order to evaluate breathing patterns.
   f. practicing reading out loud from passages of various books, changing the inflection, rate and internal emo-

tions associated with the passage.

g. Finally, but not least in the order of "practising," is a heightened awareness during moments of stress, such as in competitive events or games in which I am a coach or activity leader, to "selfishly select" the most appropriate verbal cues rather than create a constant stream of "coaching noise."

In concluding my story, I reflect upon one of Alanna's key tips. She said that the trained person who had conditioned his or her voice correctly could "feel the sound." The "experts" knew when their voice was right. My minimal experiences with a voice training program suggest that there is indeed an "art as well as a science" to correct care of the voice. The future of my voice quality will be directly related to the time and effort invested in daily practice. Regardless of my individual discipline, I am forever indebted to Alanna for providing me a chance to begin again.

The Case of Shawnee Harle,
Basketball Coach and Teacher of Physical Education

Background

In September, 1994, Shawnee Harle became the women's varsity intercollegiate basketball coach for the University of Calgary. She is the sixth in the history of the program. A native of Campbell River, B.C., Shawnee graduated from the University of Victoria where she played on two of their national championship basketball teams. She also attended the National Coaching Institute in Victoria, British Columbia, where she completed her Level IV national coaches certification program; she is two tasks short of attaining her Level V certification. She has also completed the majority of her work towards a Masters degree. Before accepting the Calgary position, Shawnee had been the Head Coach at Brandon University in Brandon, Manitoba. Prior to that experience she had been the assistant coach of the women's basketball program at the University of Victoria. In addition, she has been the Assistant Coach for Team Canada's national women's basketball program operating during the summers from 1992 to the present. She was a member of the coaching staff for Team Canada at the 1994 World Basketball Championships in Australia and the 1994 Goodwill Games in Russia. Her story, told in her voice, was taped during an interview.

The Story

I never had voice problems as a player. However, as soon as I moved into the field of coaching I started encountering a variety of difficulties, some as simple as a feeling in the evening of being "voice tired or strained" to the worse scenario of completely losing my voice. Those types of vocal difficulties have been on going for the past ten years, ever since I started as a basketball coach. Upon reflection, the vocal disorders directly relate to my coaching style, the physical environments of basketball gymnasiums, the length of the basketball season, the number of coaching sessions and games, and the level of vocal intensity that is needed to encourage and motivate the players. In most cases I am "rewarded" for the increased vocal volume, as I perceive an immediate visual feedback when the player changes the movement pattern or the action needed to be more successful. If I did not see such immediate or instant change there would not be any need for such change in the tone or intensity of my voice. I get rewarded for verbal misuse.

Specifically analyzing the previous reasons for vocal failure, I know that my major source for vocal distress, especially so very early in my coaching career, has been due to the "spirited" use of my voice. I have always been a very emotional and passionate person, especially as a coach in the use of verbal communications with my players. It has always been a big part of me which I believe reflects my personality. I have always wanted players to feel that I am practising and competing with them. I do not want them to feel that I operate only as a dictator, providing instructions or awarding punishment in disciplinary situations. I want my players to know that I am with them. Therefore, I have always felt that I had to have a strong vocal level to order to motivate and encourage them to practise and play at their highest possible level of intensity.

The second opportunity for vocal misuse is related to the environment in which I work. In all basketball situations, the majority of the training and competing occurs in gymnasiums. Thus I speak over background noises of other teams or spectators, poor acoustics related to lack of soundproofing building materials or just the distances that normally occur between the players and me as a part of the movement drills associated with the sport. Another influence that I had difficulty acknowledging was a residual vocal fatigue that carried into my practice sessions from the morning and afternoon classroom and gym activities.

During my first coaching experience, in a high school setting, I always found that the worst time was when I came home from weekend tournaments, which involved a minimum of three games, sometimes in a row. I would come back from those tournaments with a squeaky and raspy voice, and in many cases with a voice volume reduced to a mere whisper. This condition lasted for two to three days into the week following the tournaments.

However, I did not think that there was anything wrong with that vocal condition. I just accepted it, knowing that with a few day's rest the voice level would improve toward the end of the week. It was like winning and losing. It was just a part of the job. I did not worry about this condition or even consider looking for a medical opinion of any sort. Due to the nature of a short competitive season, lasting for only three or four months, in addition to only two to three practice sessions per week at the high school level, I never developed chronic vocal disorder other than those tournament weekends. There always seemed to be enough time for my voice to fully recover.

Once I started coaching at the university level as a head coach, however, everything changed. Now the season increased to at least six to seven months, with weekly practice sessions including a minimum of six sessions per week. The recovery time was reduced to only one day, with only some slight variation relative to the time of the year. In my first year at the Canadian Intercollegiate Athletic Union level (C.I.A.U.), which lasted from September to April, I was selected to be an assistant coach with the national team which practised and competed from April to August. For the first time in my life I was actively coaching basketball twelve months a year.

It was at the end of the first full year of coaching that I really started noticing major signs of voice strain, with deterioration of the volume and little power to talk higher than a whisper. Again, however, because I assumed that this was just a part of the profession, longer terms of whispering, rasping and loss of volume just became part of me. As the weakening process was gradual, I internally adjusted and became used to the change. I would come home from weekend games during the university season with a vocal level that ranged from simply terrible to nonexistent. The voice improved slightly, or to a level I deemed satisfactory, because any condition stronger than a whisper was better than a complete loss of voice.

The first time I consciously became aware my voice was deteriorating was when I talked with my family on the phone right after beginning university coaching. Because family members were not around me on a regular basis, they could more easily detect something wrong. My father was the first to point out to me that something was very wrong with my voice. I thought he was kidding. I honestly felt my voice was very good, suggesting to him that if he thought it was bad he should listen to me immediately after a weekend game.

Now completing my third year as a head coach at the C.I.A.U. level in Canada, I know that my voice recovers more slowly and to a lower level of health than it did during my first year. So it seems like the wear and tear is taking its toll. The recovery and healing process seems to leave me with a lingering rasp to my speech in addition to a reduced speaking volume. Even though such symptoms indicated the need for seeking outside medical help, I was still slow to respond.

My failure to seek external medical help may be related to coaches who were athletes, or the competitive image that we are supposed to be "tough," but I have never been very good at seeking personal help. When I am sick or when I am injured, I have always resisted turning to those authorities who could assist me. In fact, due to the intensity of making the sport experience the best for my players and the team, I probably leave areas of my own health and wellbeing at the bottom of the daily list of things to do. It is an interesting coaching paradox, because I attempt to elicit every possible external opinion in search of the best for my athletes, knowing if they are not healthy physically or mentally, they cannot play to their potential. I have always assumed that I will always be ready to coach.

A couple of critical incidents occurred this year which finally helped me realize that I needed to see someone for help. The first major realization that I needed to take action was my difficulty in recovering. I noticed practice sessions were more difficult. At one intense moment in a game this year, my players could not hear me, even though I thought I was yelling at the top of my voice.

The second incident was probably the most compelling. I was fortunate that one of my assistant coaches this year had friends who had experienced vocal disorders similar to mine. She was very persistent in making me realize that I needed to attend to this problem immediately. Her friends, who had nodule problems, were successful in returning vocal effectiveness by working in therapy with a local speech pathologist. For awhile I tended to ignore her pushing and prodding; I just could not envision when I would ever have the time to go see a specialist. Finally, at the end of the season I really had run out of "time excuses." My assistant coach, impatient with my lack of action, did all of the leg work, obtaining the therapist's name, phone number and address. She phoned the therapist and explained my situation. In simple words: it was time, I had to go!

The speech and language pathologist was Ms. Alanna McDonough at Foothills Hospital in Calgary. When I first phoned regarding an appointment, I had just barely started talking with her when she indicated that I definitely needed to meet with her immediately. I was astounded, as I felt that my voice was "great." I noted that my season had been over for two weeks, commenting that she should have heard my voice during the season.

I visited her over a period of four to five weeks, meeting twice a week for "voice lessons." I think it was like dealing with any life change habit: you first have to become aware that there is a problem before any remedies or processes can be developed to change the behavior. The sessions were very informative. As an example: who really thinks about breathing or where your pitch level should be while talking? Physical sensations, such as pushing with your diaphragm rather than using and straining your vocal cords, especially from the front or nasal part of your voice, were uniquely new pieces of information that I had never considered before.

Basically, I learned steps to use my voice more correctly and properly, emphasizing the areas to make the necessary changes in restoring vocal efficiency. The changes that must be made will be very difficult for me, as the background noises in my practice environment will always remain "busy." There will always be adjacent teams in the main gymnasium. There will always be distance between the players and me during movement drills. There will always be a need to amplify my voice at high levels for purposes of motivation and encouragement.

Those are the coaching facts of life: I cannot change them. However, I am looking at new ways in which some of those patterns can be altered so that my voice can be saved, especially since this is the career and profession that I have chosen. This new awareness has yet to be tested, as I did all of the voice training in the off-season. It will start this summer when I start working with the national team in Toronto.

I know that I have a long way to go because some serious and dedicated time has to be spent training my voice. It is very similar to the type of commitment that I ask of my players. I know that my lifestyle is not going to change much. If I am to survive as a coach, some habits will have to change. Some of the more immediate ways that I hope to concentrate upon include:

1. attempting to analyze all potential "misuse" situations that might occur in the practice environment. I will try to modify or reduce the potential impact by finding different ways to bring the team together.

2. moving in closer proximity to the players during moments of high intensity so that the pitch and volume can be reduced.

3. utilizing full breathing and pushing from the diaphragm when the pitch and volume has to be increased.

4. reducing the quantity of words and phrases by inserting key concepts.

5. paying more attention to what I am saying rather than just providing constant "coaching noise."

6. positioning myself closer to the players during moments of critical feedback.

7. sharing my vocal dilemma with my players so that they too can help me help myself. This type of dialogue can be developed at the beginning of the year, using a set of hand signals and nonverbal communication cues.

8. thinking when getting player's attention during practice and rethinking how I can reduce volume during a game. I can remember when I was a player at the University of Victoria. My coach and coaching mentor, Ms. Kathy Shields, a most successful basketball coach, had a very low coaching voice in volume, yet I always heard her as a player. She never yelled at referees or the players. Perhaps I need to consider how she was able to successfully perform.

9. working at hydrating more regularly during practice sessions. I hydrate consistently during games and have my water bottle constantly by my side. However, I seem to have difficulty remembering to bring my water bottle to the practice environment. This crucial area for improvement is a priority during the upcoming season.

10. Finally, as Alanna recommended, looking into some form of portable sound system, similar to those used by aerobic instructors. It is a new possibility that I have not explored. I am not sure of the technical implications or requirements that would be needed, nor am I certain about possible noise interference to adjacent teams.

The Case of Tim Bothwell,
Hockey Coach

Background

In September, 1994, Tim Bothwell became the men's interim varsity intercollegiate hockey coach for the University of Calgary, replacing Willy Desjardins who is currently on a two-year leave of absence to coach in Japan. Tim played many years as a minor hockey player in Canada before moving to Brown University in the United States to play four years of collegiate hockey. After graduating with a Bachelor's degree in political science and economics, he went on to play professional major and "farm team" hockey in the National Hockey League for twelve years, playing for the New York Rangers, St. Louis Blues and Hartford Whalers. In his last year as a professional hockey player, Tim was a player-coach with one of the farm teams of the Los Angeles Kings located in New Haven, Connecticut. His first "coaching only position" was for two years with the Medicine Hat Tigers of the Western Hockey League. From there he went to the International Hockey League farm team of the Los Angeles Kings located in Phoenix for two years. Then, he assumed the position at the University of Calgary. In his first year at the University, the Dinos won the Canada West Hockey Championships and were one of four national teams to participate at this year's C.I.A.U. National Championships. The following edited dialogue is his story.

The Story

I have always been a very vocal guy, whether as a player on the ice or sitting on the bench. That is how I grew up. It was a normal part of a career playing hockey. I never had any trouble with my voice or noticed that my voice was deteriorating until the last three or four years of my playing career. At that time I can remember other teammates starting to tease me about my voice. It was probably the first clue that I had that something might be wrong. Even then I really did not think the sound of my voice had changed because the vocal damage to the voice had been gradual over a long period of time.

Knowing that I would be coaching fulltime in Medicine Hat and anticipating voice difficulties, I purchased a wireless remote microphone and receiver system, similar to those used by the fitness industry's aerobic instructors. I had the idea that this equipment could be used on the ice during practice sessions. I did not purchase separate speakers as I wanted something simple and portable, figuring that the receiver could be patched into any major speaker system.

I used this system on a regular basis in Medicine Hat during practices for the full two years that I was there. The receiver was linked to the arena's public address system. The system featured a wireless microphone which was clipped to the waist of my sweat pants. The microphone had an on and off switch, to use when the players were skating over the entire ice surface. This technology was to be extremely valuable. It was easy to use my normal speaking voice, even if the players were at the opposite end of the ice. I felt less tension in "forcing" my voice when I needed to encourage or motivate.

Even with the wireless microphone system, I still had constant voice problems after weekend games. The weekend games involved three games in a three night period. On Monday morning there was a noticeable tone difference, because the power and volume was reduced to a whisper. In fact, that was probably the first time that I really accepted that I had voice problems.

When I coached in Phoenix, I attempted to continue using the wireless system. However, the system was not used as consistently as in Medicine Hat. Some of the difficulties involved the patching of the two different systems. I also had problems with the microphone because the on and off switch operation was faulty. A greater problem involved the technical setup prior to each practice. The arena's staff had to insure that the various cords and switches were set in place prior to my arrival on the ice. Many times I was ready to start a practice and the system would not be in place. As a coach, practice time is valuable, so I would continue without the sound system. I could never seem to find the consistency in Phoenix which would have provided technological support for my voice.

When I moved to Calgary, I encountered new challenges in using my wireless system. The Olympic Oval is unlike any other arena that I have ever worked in. One has to see it to appreciate the size and the use by other groups. There are two hockey rinks surrounded by a four hundred meter speed skating track. In addition to the size of the facility, which alone dwarfs most vocal projections, the associated ambient noise in the Oval is tremendous. All three venues are actively used throughout the day with athletes or teams of various ice disciplines training and competing. In addition to community groups participating in free skating at various times of the day, there is the sound of music and announcements from the main speaker system, plus the noise of the Zamboni ice machines preparing ice surfaces. It was obvious that I definitely needed some sort of sound system to protect what voice I had left.

However, whenever I patched my wireless system into the main speakers at the Oval it eliminated the entire sound system for all other user groups. Because of the greater needs of having the main speaker system available for the entire facility, I attempted to use a portable system. That system had very small speakers, limiting the clarity and power. Sometimes I could not hear myself talking to the players. In effect, I never was quite sure if they were understanding what the "coaching message" was due to the lack of power or quality of the sound. I also encountered setup difficulties similar to Phoenix.

After using a speaking system, it is very frustrating to not to have an adequate system on a consistent basis, or to have difficulties at the start of a practice so that I never know if the unit is in place and ready to go. Many of the practice planning sessions are related to how I can communicate with the guys. If they are spread out all over the ice, I need to be able to make contact with them.

I am sure that this type of frustration only adds additional tension to my mindset which then transmits a message to my vocal area, knowing that I will have to push even harder to get my verbal instructions and information out to the players. As an example, without the system, I can be talking to the guys within a ten foot circle but they have a hard time hearing me.

In conjunction with the purchase of the remote system, I also went to see a voice therapist in Medicine Hat. She talked about voice placement, "warming-up" the voice, using different locations of vocal expression within the voice cavity and developing proper breath support that can be developed while under tension or above normal speaking volumes. She provided me with inhalation and exhalation exercises associated with various sounds, words and phrases.

However, I have not practiced the exercises on a consistent basis since those sessions. I guess it is like regular physical exercise: unless one plans for it one never seems to have the time. I am certainly more aware now of certain situations in which my voice is being misused. As an example, I know that during game situations, when a vocal projection is going to have to be made, proper breath support is definitely needed. As of yet I have not had much success in changing this vocal misuse pattern, but I am working on it.

There are some suggestions, however, that the therapist offered that I have consistently incorporated into my daily coaching regimen. The list includes efforts:

1. to hydrate on a consistent basis with water before and during a game.

2. to eliminate coffee prior to and during a game. The caffeine has a tendency to dry out the vocal cords.

3. to chew sugarless gum or a succulent type of candy constantly throughout a game.

4. to be more selective in verbal information delivered to the players. This solution might be a positive concept, regardless of vocal limitations. Sometimes "coach noise" becomes more of a nervous habit rather than a delivery of critical or quality information. Players can become used to the general noise and in some cases "tune out." With selective vocal information, the listening ability of the players might improve. In addition, I save my voice for those really critical moments, during both the practice session and the game, when the encouragement, motivation and technical information is really needed.

Even with all my vocal difficulties, I have yet to fully lose my voice at any point in my coaching career although I anticipate that this might be a logical possibility sometime in the future. Since moving to the college level I have noticed less strain and soreness, probably because there are only two games per week. Both are usually held on weekends, so there is a week of rest in between.

As a side note, my father, the former Archbishop of Ontario for the Anglican Church, had some voice problems during the last five years of his service to the Church. He retired about four years ago. Because of the nature of the work, he constantly used his voice in a variety of ways on a daily basis throughout the year. There really were no rest periods. I am not sure if he encountered voice problems during his early career with the Church. However, on several occasions during the later years he would completely lose his voice. The condition was diagnosed as acute laryngitis. The loss of the voice would last three or four days. He recovered with no noticeable vocal afflictions, such as a whisper or weak voice.

I am not sure if the problems he experienced were a result of long term overuse in conjunction with the aging process or just a unique moment in time for him. Nevertheless, it is something that I am going to have to be aware of as I get older, because I already have experienced major voice problems. My life journey is only approaching a midpoint; I turn forty this month. I will have to work at avoiding further vocal misuse situations in my coaching career and life if I am to reduce my own voice failures in the future.

Physical Education Teacher Case Studies

Background

The following case study examples were derived from teachers operating in a physical education or athletic program in a elementary, junior or senior high school in Calgary. The teachers were surveyed regarding vocal difficulties encountered during the school year in the teaching and coaching of physical activities. I believe they represent only a "snapshot" of what is really happening to their colleagues throughout

North America who have had similar voice problems. As did the three coaches in the previous case studies, most think they do not have a "real problem." Their stories suggest that a teacher preparation and professional development day in-service related to proper voice training and care is a necessity.

Francine's Story

Grade Level: Years 4-10

Teaching Experience: 5 years

Voice Problems:

Every year I lose my voice completely, usually around October and again during the spring. Numerous times during the school year I have very bad sore throats.

My Solutions:

1. to talk less.

2. to use a lower tone of voice.

3. to give most of the instructions at the beginning of the gym class.

4. to use a lot of nonverbal signals.

Gerri's Story

Grade Level: E.C.S. to Grade 6

Teaching Experience: 20 years

Voice Problems:

Over the last ten years or so, especially at the beginning and the end of the school year (high stress times) my voice slowly fades until I have to take three or four days off just to rest it. My throat is not sore – it is just gone. I feel tired when I try to talk.

My Solutions:

1. to use lots of body language. My students help me describe and develop fun hand signals.

2. to use a mini-microphone on my shirt. My voice projects out of six speakers. It is especially valuable when I do the dance unit with music.

3. to call the students closer to me prior to issuing instructions.

4. to choose students to convey my message, letting them be "my voice."

5. to flick the lights on and off in the change room to let the students know it is time to go rather than yelling.

6. to use ancillary devices such as the traditional whistle or tambourine to let them know when to stop or go.

7. to use charts containing tasks to be done.

Tom's Story

Grade Level: Years 5-7 and University

Teaching Experience: 21 years

Voice Problems:

I lose my voice in many instances during coaching, especially in hockey arenas.

My Solutions:

1. to use my whistle for stop/go commands.

2. to gather my players close to me, like a huddle, having them face me when I talk.

3. to develop gamelike drills that run by themselves. This strategy allows me to talk with one player at a time instead of continually keeping the drill going.

4. to identify one theme and focus on it at the start of the gym period or practice session, reminding myself of the theme throughout to save my voice.

Michele's Story

Grade Level: Six

Teaching Experience: 8 years

Voice Problems:

I have a deeper voice than do most females. My voice often goes hoarse after an active day of teaching in the gym or on the field outside. It is often raspy or rough. I was also a lifeguard for eight years which contributed to my voice difficuties. I have heard that I may have "vocal nodules" or related damage to my vocal cords, but I have never had a doctor's assessment.

My Solutions:

1. to use hand and whistle signals.

2. to use student leaders to help convey my message.

3. to use charts on the walls. Using charts outside has not always been practical, however, because of weather and a lack of appropriate places to put the charts.

James' Story

Grade Level: Years 10-12

Teaching Experience: 12 years

Voice Problems:

I lose my voice in many instances during special event time periods such as the start of school, Christmas, tournament weekends, play-offs, and especially when we move outdoors to the field activities. Some of the irritations that have caused me vocal difficulty include a reduction of vocal power, almost to a whisper, hoarseness, a gravelly sound that remains with me in normal conversation and a general state of fatigue at the end of the day and week. Sometimes I just do not want to talk when I leave school.

My Solutions:

1. to explain to each class that I have voice problems, especially toward the end of the day. I have them work with me in helping me.

2. to carry a reasonably large white board for field activities that I can carry with me to write some of the more general instructions or stations.

3. to carry a portable "game clock" to signify when a drill session is ending. This is especially effective during station drills.

4. to use a bullhorn. However, except for general commands, I find it hard to use on a personal basis. It reminds me too much of a military situation rather than one involved with teaching.

Marjolaine's Story

Grade Level:	Grades 7-9
Teaching Experience:	14 years

Voice Problems:

I "almost" lose my voice during the first few weeks of teaching every year. Even during the rest of the year, regardless of how careful I am during classes to avoid straining my voice, I find that by Friday a certain amount of hoarseness and soreness has developed.

My Solutions:

1. to use a fair number of hand signals or general body language to direct activity.

2. to have my students direct activity or provide "start/stop" instructions.

3. to use a countdown, fairly loudly, but only three sounds: "1-2-3".

4. to gather five to ten students and ask them to sit down close by me. I start providing instructions in a low voice. Then the rest of the students outside of this group usually stop and redirect their attention towards this group.

Diane's Story

Grade Level:	Years 1-6
Teaching Experience:	13 years

Voice Problems:

I can feel a strain on my vocal chords when speaking at any time, soft or loud. I feel a loss of vocal power. I am constantly clearing my throat as if there is a "coating" on my vocal chord.

My Solutions:

1. to use a mixture of robitussin and liquid calcium obtained from a pharmacist. I use it when needed.

2. to use a microphone in the gym at all times, especially when my voice gets bad.

3. to refrain from cheering or issuing coaching instructions loudly when watching or supervising games or sporting activities.

4. to talk or laugh in a *low* tone, trying not to raise the pitch of the voice.

Conclusions

After listening to these "coaching voices," it seems obvious that:

1. The physical environment is not conducive to protecting the coaching voice. Whether it is the size of the facility or playing field, the variety of temperatures, the competing noises or the distance between athletes or students during activity, there will be a need for voice projection even for the most basic communications. Because there seems to be a need for a "heightened vocal volume" for purposes of motivation, encouragement and critical feedback, the additional strain and potential misuse will be a constant threat. Therefore, environmental alternatives for communicating should be developed. These strategies involve electronic technology for amplifying the voice, alarm systems indicating the start/stop sequencing such as using the scoreboard buzzer or colored lights such as the goal light in the hockey rink to signify a meeting with the coach is required.

2. The method and style of communicating, especially during practice sessions, should be reviewed and adjusted. The development of a variety of hand and body

nonverbal cues and signals, squad meetings that are "up close and personal," and portable white boards or bulletin boards for fundamental information are samples of what can be developed to save the coach's voice. Perhaps sharing with one's players the limitations of the voice during practice sessions would assist players to "help the coach." Saving the coach's voice for the game can become as important a team mission as competing.

3. Practice hydrating during practices and games. Players hydrate to replace lost internal body fluids during exercise. Coaches also need to keep their voices from drying out.

4. During competitive moments, especially those with a high degree of stress, the coach should consider the selection of phrases and voice projection level carefully. Coaching is an art under stress, meaning that "what one sees on the playing field" and how one "responds vocally" is usually an emotional reaction. However, with practice, it might be possible for the coach to practice using proper breath support during simple and effective "vocal cues," progressing to more emotional responses, without "losing it." Then, in a game situation, much as in the players' practice drills, the coach might have a better chance of using the coaching voice mor correctly and effectively.

5. It is important to develop and implement the study of caring for the voice, including protection and enhancement techniques, into various teacher preparation programs. Professional sport coaches also need voice care training.

6. Finally, but not last in my conclusions, is the recommendation that all coaches and teachers in the field of physical activity who encourage their athletes to "play hard" and "be tough," modify those cliches with regard to the care of their own voice. The preferred coaching voice clichés might be "speak well" and "take care." The voice is a key ingredient to success in our profession. In addition to encouraging and motivating players to do their best, we must coach ourselves to

ers to do their best, we must coach ourselves to develop "voice excellence."

DONALD MCGAVERN, M.Sc., is Manager of Aquatics and a member of the Faculty of Kinesology at the University of Calgary. Within this chapter, he summarized relevant career achievements, using his experiences as a case study of someone who eventually was diagnosed with a "chronic vocal disorder."

CHAPTER 3
Working to Develop the Voice
Janine Pearson and Kelly McEvenue

Introduction – Janine Pearson

Teachers need to identify themselves as "professional voice users," as people whose job and livelihood relies upon the ability to impart information through the use of their voice. Like actors, teachers also have an audience, their students, to whom they desire to impart knowledge. In contrast, however, actors study voice and movement in depth throughout their performing lives. Regretfully, practical voice training and the development of oral skills are rarely emphasized in teacher education, leaving teachers with an insufficient knowledge of how to use their voices.

This situation was not always the case. When my grandmother trained as a teacher in the early 1900s, a large part of her training involved speech and elocution, singing and the recitation of poetry and prose. As we quickly approach the twenty-first century we can easily argue that we have left that time far behind. After all, who's ever heard of speech and elocution? Isn't that something that is saved for the local high school's production of *My Fair Lady* – and more specifically for the actor playing Henry Higgins. Doesn't it conjure up the thought of proper speech and, more to the point, proper *British* speech? As for singing, isn't this training something that belongs to the music teacher? Can you imagine or remember the days when singing was as natural as speaking, when people used their voices in an open and extended way? There was a time when people passed on their stories through song, when family history or political experience was presented through music and words. People spoke for the sheer enjoyment of speaking poetry aloud! These practices disappeared during my time at school. However, my grandmother could recite poems and narrative passages from memory, passages which she had learned at school or in training. These words never left her. They were always on the tip of her tongue. They were always available to her imagination and ours.

The further we are distanced from an oral tradition, the more our bodies and voices look for ways to return. Our voices want to be open and expressive. After all, most of us have experienced these feelings at one time in our lives – during childhood. As a child I remember feeling embarrassed when my mother would report that she'd heard me playing while she was working in her kitchen and I was out in the barn! How could she hear me? Obviously I was much too loud. I thought this behavior to be a very unladylike attribute and worked hard to create a mild mannered voice befitting the young girl I wished to be. By the time I was on stage in university, however, my voice teacher was telling me that I couldn't be heard at the back of the theatre.

Whether this change is inevitable or not is debatable. Voice teachers have talked about the problem for years. Theatre directors moan about actors whose voices and bodies are weak. Meanwhile, voice scientists and language pathologists have become fascinated with the few cultures in the world that seem to be sheltered from this vocal inhibition. Their studies reveal what teachers and directors have always known: we need to develop an awareness of ourselves, more specifically, of our bodies and voices.

When I began as a Voice Coach for the Stratford Festival (Stratford, Ontario) I was asked by the Education Coordinator in Spring, 1990, to speak to a group of visiting teachers about *the voice*. I was surprised, and somewhat shocked, when instead of lecturing to this group I found myself listening to their concerns: "I am hoarse every September"; "I don't like the sound of my voice in the classroom"; "I feel as though I am always screaming at my kids"; "By the time I get home, after a day of teaching, I feel as though I haven't got enough voice left to speak to my own family"; "I used to sing in the church choir, but I can't anymore. My voice is just too tired." A feeling of frustration permeated that room. What could they do? Or more to the point, what hadn't they done? The problem was simple: they needed to rediscover their own voices – how to use them, how to protect them and most of all how to enjoy them in communication.

This experience made such an impression that I wondered if there wasn't something that we could do to help these professionals. They could benefit from the skills we use in the theatre. Working in cooperation with the company's Alexander Technique Coach, Kelly McEvenue, we began the Voice Care and Development Workshops for Teachers as part of the Summer Institute at the Stratford Festival, and since then have been helping teachers in facilitating a freer use of their voices by incorporating practical voice work with the Alexander Technique. We have been delighted and enthused by the opportunity of offering our work to professional teachers.

Our teaching experience has been primarily with performing artists, actors, singers and musicians who want to understand the freedom and flexibility of the body and voice as necessary tools in expressing their art form. We have been curious to learn about the needs and vocal problems of teachers who rely on their own physical energy to communicate to students. Like an actor, their bodies are instruments of expression. However, they rarely hear any applause for a job well done.

In this chapter, Kelly and I present a clear process by which a richer understanding of one's own voice is possible. It is our desire to demystify "the voice" and examine how it works in a practical, not a theoretical, way. This process involves an understanding of how the body works and its relation to the use and expression of the voice. We begin with a profile of the Alexander Technique; then we offer suggestions for practising relaxation, breathing and stretches. We provide exercises that help connect sound to the body and develop vocal range and focus. After these warm ups we suggest tongue twisters and poetry to facilitate a connection between voice and language.

The Alexander Technique – Kelly McEvenue

Frederick Matthias Alexander was a Tasmanian actor and orator who developed the Alexander Technique in Australia at the turn of the last century. Ironically, he made his discovery about the organization and co-ordination of the body as a

Figure 1: Head-Neck Relationship

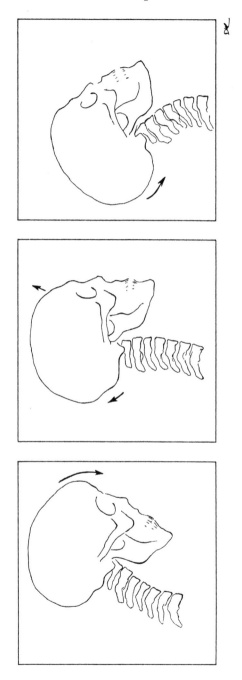

result of continually losing his voice. He was a great lover of Shakespeare and enjoyed the 19th century practice of recitation. To lose his voice was to deny him his greatest pleasure and his livelihood. With an actor's passion and a talent for observing human character, he set out to understand his vocal problem by painstakingly examining the manner in which he used his body when he produced his voice. He observed the three dimensional view of his body by surrounding himself with mirrors. He noted that when he began to speak, he would gasp for breath while at the same time contracting his head back and down onto his spine. This movement locked his body into a set posture, creating tension throughout his neck, torso and legs. Thus, his entire organism was affected by this one contracting movement. All this tension was created just so he could begin to breathe and communicate! Alexander realized that the habitual and excessive downward pressure of his head onto his body restricted his natural flexibility and thereby interfered with his vocal instrument. He noticed this pattern would occur every time he began to speak.

Alexander decided he had to STOP this habitual response. Once he inhibited or stopped this habit of contraction, he could then consider making a change. He needed to reorganize the head and neck relationship if he was ever to release all the downward pressure in his body. He stopped (inhibited) the habitual pattern and then applied the conscious thought, "allow my neck to be free, to allow my head to move forward and up, to allow my back to lengthen and widen." Eureka! Through this thinking process he was able to redirect his old movement pattern, thereby releasing the pressure in his neck and freeing his voice.

Here, the discovery and the development of a technique are summarized in a few words, when in fact it took Alexander years of scientific experimentation. Alexander worked on his own until his brother, A. R. Alexander, became involved in developing what is now called "The Alexander Technique." What was and is so unique in this work is that a student can learn to apply conscious thinking to redirect the misuse of the body into a more flexible and free state of being. Scientists call this motion of the body "the primary control." We can see the primary control in any animal's movement: be that a giraffe running with its head moving in a forward and upward direction or in the development of a toddler learning to walk. Alexander spent his lifetime studying human functioning and developing the application of his discovery in human movement. Learning to consciously direct "the primary control" of our bodies is the basic concept of the Alexander Technique.

All sorts of people other than performing artists have benefitted from lessons with a certified Alexander Teacher: people with a variety of physical problems including sciatica, poor posture, breathing difficulties, whip lash, headaches and a variety of stress-related problems. The Alexander teacher can objectively identify habits of misuse in the student, habits which are difficult to discern on one's own. More importantly, the teacher gives the student a "hands on" experience, providing a kinesthetic stimulus or direction to the student's head and neck, thereby introducing the new redirection of the student's coordination and encouraging the primary control to bring the body into balance. The work can be taught in private lessons or in group classes.

Relaxation – Janine Pearson

There has been a great deal written about relaxation during the past decade. The hectic pace of our daily lives has been instrumental in creating an entirely new industry promoting the art of relaxation and its benefits. Therapists within a wide variety of fields use relaxation as a means to help people get in touch with their bodies and their emotions. Many doctors recommend relaxation for patients with high blood pressure, heart problems and other stress-related diseases. For those with severe health problems, who are forced to use daily relaxation techniques, they can be a life-changing experience. They may also be used as a form of deep meditation and prayer, a method of enabling a spiritual experience. In its relationship to the Alexander Technique and voice work, however, relaxation plays a very specific role. Through the use of relaxation we begin to differentiate between the quality of our muscular tension as opposed to the quantity of muscular tension that we engage in our bodies and voices when we communicate. We need to discern the difference between the tension required to keep our bodies in the upright position and the kind of tension that prevents or inhibits us from using our bodies and voices to their full extent. We need to understand that unnecessary physical tension affects the voice in many adverse ways. For example, people experiencing excess tension in the head, neck and shoulder areas may: (1) speak at a higher vocal pitch, which lacks the full resonance of tone or (2) use strained articulation, which creates discomfort in their jaw. This habitual jaw tension, in turn, might cause headaches or nightly grinding of the teeth. (3) develop a habitually stiff neck, which eventually impedes the easy cycle of the breath. This strain may be observed through an audible inhalation in some people.

Equally unnecessary tension in the lower back or abdominal area also inhibits the full movement of the breath and interferes with support of the voice. Our mothers' generation will remember the days of girdles and corsets. These so-called garments of feminine beauty helped to create the ever delicate and lightly voiced personalities that were as unnatural as the material with which they themselves were made. Corsets, girdles and belts were cinched so tight that breathing became a thought and not an actuality. Is it any wonder then that women had the reputation of being weak, fragile and prone to unpredictable spells of fainting?

Try the simple relaxation exercise that follows. Initially, you could set aside twenty minutes for this exercise. However, if you have never done relaxation before you might want to give yourself a little longer. At the beginning, people get discouraged. They panic when they think of how long it takes to accomplish the desired state of ease. But do not get discouraged. It will not always take twenty minutes to accomplish the desired results. It's like any new skill on which you work: it takes longer at the beginning. People who have been doing it for years can find that place of ease in a single breath.

Begin by lying on your back with a pillow under your head and a second pillow under your knees. Lie on a surface which is not too hard (i.e., a hardwood floor), but do not lie on a surface which is too soft (i.e., your bed) unless you want to sleep! Take your shoes off. You might want to cover yourself with a blanket. Some people find that, as they begin to relax, their body temperature falls. It is better to have a blanket handy than to have to stop the exercise in order to go and get one. You might want to do this exercise while listening to your favorite piece of music, something that you find restful and easy.

Before you begin, read the exercise through to completion, familiarizing yourself with each of the steps. In doing so, you will be able to concentrate fully on the exercise at hand and not be continually distracted, having to break your focus by going back and forth to and from the directions. As you talk yourself through this exercise initially, you may want to have your eyes closed. Do what makes you feel comfortable. For many people, beginning with their eyes closed is an easy way of blocking out the world and all of its overstimulation. However, I encourage you, at some point, to do this exercise with your eyes open. Experience the easing in the body while your mind is alert and able to focus clearly. After all, relaxation need not be the first step on the way to sleep.

Begin by sending a direction (in the form of a request) to your <u>feet</u>, telling them to soften and release. You will need to constantly remind yourself to breathe comfortably and deeply without pushing. Continue the journey upwards from your feet towards your <u>ankles</u>. This progression can be as detailed or as specific as your time permits. From the ankles, proceed to the <u>calves of the legs,</u> and then to the <u>thighs</u>. As you direct the legs to soften you think specifically about all of the muscles.

Continue to the <u>lower abdominal area;</u> to the <u>buttocks</u> and <u>belly</u> (or what I affectionately refer to as the "bowl"). Once you are in this area you begin the journey up the spine. Travel one vertebra at a time, giving yourself the opportunity to picture the spaces between each vertebrae and thinking of the muscles in the back as softening and widening as they melt into the floor. Allow your rib cage to soften and widen. Once again, remind yourself to breathe. If you carry a great deal of tension in your upper body you may want to go more slowly over this particular area. Directing the sternum (breast *bone) to soften and relax will, in turn, enable the shoulders to release and fall towards the floor.*

As you think about the muscles in the top and back of the neck (which is actually the top of the spine), allow them to soften as well. This relaxation facilitates the release of your very heavy head into the pillow. Imagine that you don't have to work to hold your head up in this position. Let the pillow do that. Breathe as deeply and with as much ease as possible. If you can contact the weight of your own head and release it into the pillow you will find that the muscles in your neck will begin to soften and release also. The release of these muscles is of the utmost importance as they directly affect the free movement of the vocal mechanism (the larynx).

Finally, but most important, allow the muscles of the face to release – the forehead, the eyes, the cheeks, the nose, the upper lip, the jaw, the tongue, the bottom lip and the front of the neck. Breathe. Allow the weight of your body to spread into the floor with an ease and lightness. Observe the weight of your own body and breath. Does it feel light and energized or do you feel as though you could sleep for a thousand years? Regardless of how you feel, try not to impose any "shoulds" upon your state. Continue to breathe as you allow your mind to be active. Rest in this position until you feel it is appropriate to slowly get up.

Warning: some people may experience a slight dizziness if they attempt to get up too quickly. Once you are on your feet this is a perfect moment to ask yourself if your breathing pattern or location of your breath has changed. For example, after relaxation many people discover that their breathing pattern is slower, easier, and perhaps even deeper.

It's important to realize that to use relaxation as a tool everyone will need to execute it somewhat differently. For instance, some people want to use imagery, and others will not. You may want to imagine your body being drained of its unnecessary tension. You may want to think about lying on a beach and being warmed from head to foot by an non-inva-

Figure 2: Sitting in a Chair

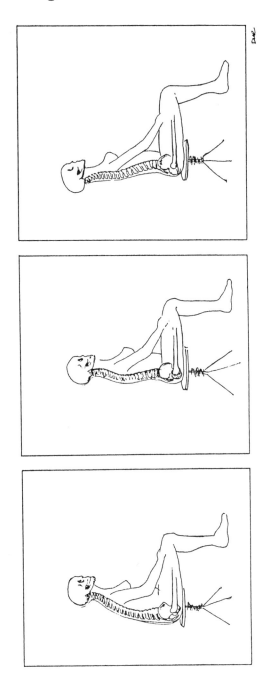

sive sun. In the end, whether you work with your eyes open or closed, with imaging or without, it doesn't matter. Whatever process you use, the important thing is that you learn to use direction: the ability to dialogue with your body.

Breath – Janine Pearson

Without breath there is no sound and, taken to the extreme, no life. To begin, we need to understand that the basic principles of relaxation and a balanced alignment assist in enabling an efficient and effective pattern of breath. Secondly, we need to recognize that this efficient and effective pattern is not unfamiliar. At birth, we experience a pattern of breath that is free, full and sustained with the greatest of ease. As we grow and mature, however, we learn through numerous physical and emotional experiences to inhibit this natural pattern. This kind of inhibition disallows many communicators from supporting their voices with the full extent of their breath. In comparison, babies are able to scream for hours on end at an excruciatingly high pitch with no apparent signs of fatigue; an adult may experience vocal strain after a couple hours of engaging conversation. This natural pattern of breath is not something that need deteriorate with age. With a little conscious thought, we, as adults, are capable of engaging our "natural and inherent breath;" thereby accessing our full potential as physical and emotional communicators.

Encouraging and reinforcing our own natural pattern of breath is often not as difficult as we may think. Unlike the relaxation exercise, this one is done sitting in a chair with your eyes open. Therefore, it is possible to read the directions as you go.

Sit in a straight chair. That is, one with a flat seat, not cushioned, with a straight back. Place both your feet flat on the floor with your legs comfortably apart. Sit away from the back of the chair. Make sure you are sitting on your ischium (commonly known as your sitting bones) and have a sense of the spine travelling up from its base to the very top of the occipital joint, between the ears, inside the skull. Allow your shoulders to relax into whatever position they please, but do not try and "set"

Figure 3: Thoracic Cavity and Vocal Apparatus

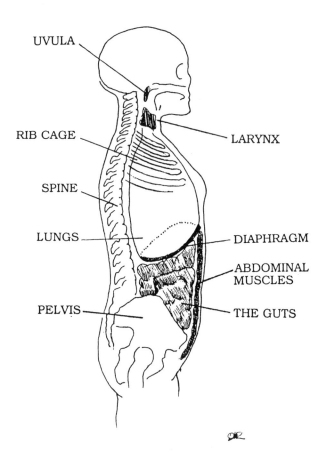

them. Allow yourself to breathe deeply and with ease. Do not push your breath at any point. Respect the natural pattern of the breath (the inhalation, the exhalation and the resting time) and listen.

Check the following areas of your body. Observe yourself physically as you breathe. After all, breath is a full-bodied experience.

- Do you experience any excess strain in the muscles of the neck and jaw? This tension may be observed by the jaw jutting forward as the head is pulled slightly back and down. This contracted position may cause unnecessary tension in the larynx resulting in an audible gasp during inhalation. In extreme cases, during moments of heightened communication, you may actually observe these neck muscles tightening and protruding as the individual's face begins to turn red!

- Are your shoulders set or held tightly in position? The most commonly held position is back and down in an attempt to achieve what we think is the square-shouldered look pertaining to good posture.

- Do you experience tightness in your upper chest? This tension may be observed with the chest rising and falling on each breath.

- Is your rib cage frozen or locked into a fixed position? A lack of flexibility in the rib cage, in particular the bottom part of the rib cage, often prevents the speaker from experiencing the full movement of the breath. It is the base of the rib cage (ribs 7 through 12) which has the most potential for movement.

- Do you push the muscles of the lower abdominal wall down and out in an attempt to breathe down into the diaphragm or, in contrast, do you believe that your stomach needs to be constantly pulled in?

If you experience any of these tensions, offer the following directions to your body as an alternative:

- Allow the neck to be free as the head travels forward and up into space. Allow the jaw to relax. That is, do not clench your teeth together, but rather allow your jaw to drop slightly open while relaxing the tongue. Allow the muscles of the neck to be soft during both the inhalation and exhalation, enabling an easy and inaudible breath.

- Allow your shoulders to drop into a relaxed position even if you feel they may be somewhat rounded. Any holding in this area may stop the breath completely. If it is difficult for you to identify a relaxed position – slowly breathe in as you bring your shoulders up towards your ears. Hold your breath and your shoulders as tightly as possible. When you can hold your breath no longer, release the breath while at the same time releasing your shoulders, letting them fall where they will. If you feel that your shoulders have found a new position do not adjust them. It is important to observe that easy and relaxed shoulders contribute to sustaining the freedom you previously discovered in the muscles of the neck and jaw.

- Allow the upper chest to be easy in its movement. Do not feel that you need to grab the air during inhalation by pulling the chest up and out. In contrast, allow your upper chest to move gently and easily. Know that the movement of your natural breath drops below your chest and down into your "bowl."

- Place your hands on the bottom and sides of your rib cage. As you breathe in allow your ribs to move gently out and upward. Do not push this movement. It is very slight, but active. Allow them to return to a more relaxed position on the exhalation. Once you have established this movement and feel confident, allow your hands to drop from this position and observe if it is possible to continue this movement gently and with ease. Remember not to push.

• If we know nothing else about the breath, we have heard about "breathing from the diaphragm." We may have no idea what this phrase means, but it is this movement that people most often exaggerate. It is important to understand that one cannot actually feel the movement of the diaphragm; rather we feel the movement of the breath in the lower abdomen as a result of the diaphragm's contraction. Therefore, do not think that you must push the diaphragm muscle rigidly down, forcing the lower abdominal wall to extend as if you were "with child." Yes, as we inhale the diaphragm does indeed contract downwards as the rib cage expands out and upwards enabling us to feel the full three-dimensional movement of the breath. But this happens naturally – if we can stay out of the way!

In contrast to this unsightly abdominal extension we see many individuals, men and women alike, who are so afraid of revealing their wonderfully round bellies that they live in a constant state of lower abdominal contraction. That is, they never allow the diaphragm and the muscles of the lower abdominal wall to release. This posture is most commonly observed at the beginning of every bathing suit season! Unfortunately, similar to the push down and out, this push is merely in the opposite direction; that is, in and up. Regardless of the direction, the movement is pushed and results in the same vocal restrictions. Therefore, despite your habit, allow these muscles to release as you inhale, enabling the breath to gently enter the body as opposed to being pulled or sucked in. The lower abdominal wall will move ever so gently out and down; not just in the front, but also at the sides and in the back. And likewise, as you exhale, allow the musculature to gently move in and up towards the spine.

The most common difficulty experienced when observing our breath is that we may become self-conscious; we may believe that our breath was working efficiently until we started to consciously think about it. I would encourage you, however, to persist in the exercise. It is the experience of understanding one's own breath during moments of self-discovery and observation that enables speakers to use their breath in active and heightened moments of communication such as teaching or performing.

Physical and Vocal Warm-up –

Janine Pearson & Kelly McEvenue

Before overcoming some of the vocal problems expressed by teachers, we need to expand our knowledge of the body, from basic anatomy to simple stretching and warming up. The professionals we encounter in our workshops have very little awareness that the tension and posture in their bodies is in any way involved in communication.

We believe it is important to introduce teachers to the concept of a warm-up, similar to the one an actor uses to prepare for the performance of a play. A warm-up is designed to prepare the performer's mind, voice and body for the demands of communicating to an audience. We want to find in the body and voice the support and readiness to work. However, it is not a "workout" which serves to challenge fitness and endurance. This type of preparation would do nothing but exhaust the performer's energy prior to the play! When we work out or perform some movement that we think will strengthen or enhance our fitness, we may tend to try too hard and feel that pushing and straining are doing the job well. Instead we cause the body to function with greater tension, decreasing our flexibility. There has been an over-zealous approach to fitness where people tend to over stretch and tighten the musculature. We can thank Arnold Schwartzenegger and Jane Fonda for creating this body culture of strain and excess during the 1980s.

In contrast to this pumped up approach, we need to gently prepare the body and the mind through the connection of breath with movement, thereby encouraging flexibility, blood circulation and alertness. We need to look at the *quality* of movement to understand its ease and fluidity. We delight in the grace and agility of wonderful movers such as Fred Astaire, Michael Jordan and Ray Bolger (the Scarecrow in *The Wizard of Oz*). Their movement appears effortless and tension-free. It is. We are observing their primary control in action, which allows their skeletal muscular system to lengthen and widen efficiently so their coordination has flexibility and control. We may never be called on to dance or play basketball professionally. However, we can still use our thinking to engage our primary control to help us in the movement challenges of our daily lives.

If you have never focused on this kind of work before, we would suggest that you work your way through the following sections, one at a time, until you feel confident with the material and have a sense of having made the work your own. Do not leave the exercises until the last minute in your morning routine – they won't work. For many teachers the day begins very early and the thought of setting aside an extra thirty minutes to stretch and hum is absolutely implausible. Remember this approach to voice is not about imposing restrictions and rigid routines, but about discovery and learning. Therefore, set aside as much time as you can afford – perhaps five or ten minutes to begin. As you experience the changes in your body, voice and the mental preparation to your day, you will find that this personal time becomes longer as you begin to bask in the knowledge that you're worth every minute!

Stretching

Lie on your back on a rug or a mat. Allow your back to be supported by the mat. Relax and breathe for a moment as you check through the basic anatomy of your body, noticing your feet, leg joints, pelvis, abdomen, rib cage, shoulder girdle, up the spine to the head. Notice how much pressure and contact the different sides or areas of your body make with the mat. Notice your legs. Do they organize out of the pelvis in the same manner? That is, do they both contact the mat in exactly the same places or does one have a greater turn out than

Figure 4: Semi-Supine Position

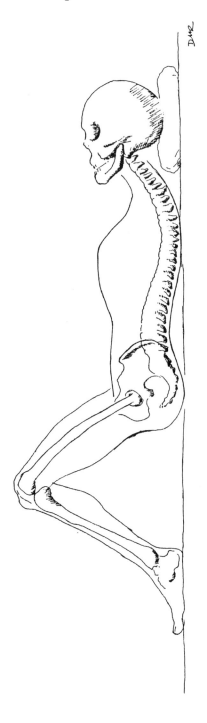

the other? How much of your back and spine contact the
mat? What about your head, neck and shoulder area?
Is there any contraction in this area? Can you sense the
size of your head? Think of the three-dimensional aspect of your limbs and torso. Draw your knees up so
that your feet are flat on the floor. This is called the
semi-supine position. Place a book or two (about an inch
in thickness) under the head to support it forward of the
spine. As the diagram indicates, notice the skeletal relationship of the head to the spine, the length of the spine,
the organization of the legs into the hip joint and the
placement of the feet on the floor. Now that your feet are
flat on the floor check through your body again, noticing
any changes where your back contacts the mat.

Place your hands underneath the back of your head. Do
not place the fingers on the neck, but on the back of the
skull. Support the weight of the head in your hands as
you curl your head and neck forward so that you look
between your knees. You should feel the heavy weight
of the head as well as the neck muscles stretching from
between the shoulder blades. Gently bring the head
back to the books and observe if there has been any
change in the relationship of your head and neck. Allow
your fingers to lead your arms up towards the ceiling.
Admire the dexterity of your fingers and the jointed
movement in your wrists and elbows. Wave them about
in space. Let one hand travel to support the weight of
the arm making contact at the joint of the wrist. Gently
pull the arm directly up towards the ceiling. You will feel
this action move the shoulder joint off the floor. When allowing the shoulder to release back to the floor, sense
the elasticity of the arm muscles. Let the arm go back to
the mat or to its neutral position before you do this
again with the other arm. Explore the range of movement and the volume of the arms and their extension
out of the back before you return them to their resting position.

Now explore the organization and range of movement in
the legs. Start by supporting the back of one of your
thighs with both hands, and encourage the weight of

the leg forward towards the torso. You will likely sense the sitting bones at the bottom of the pelvis roll off the mat. Think of allowing them to roll back to the mat even though the back of your leg has stretched forward. Relax for a moment and breathe. Breath is the fuel that will help the release and extension of the leg. Let your foot and lower leg stretch towards the ceiling. Let's not get balletic about this movement. Continue to support the weight of the leg and fuel the stretch with breath. Release the lower leg and increase the stretch of the thigh towards the torso. Again, let the foot travel up towards the ceiling and explore the ankle joint and the dexterity of the foot. Lower the leg back to the mat. Now cradle both thighs and gently bring your knees to your chest. Release. Repeat the sequence with the other leg. Remember to move gently.

Once you've completed the sequence, bring both legs to your chest. Let both feet reach up towards the ceiling and give your legs a shake. At the same time, allow your fingers to lead your arms up towards the ceiling and gently shake. Notice that in this position only your back is on the mat. Observe how your limbs organize away from the torso. We call this position, "Diapering the baby." As you release your limbs back onto the mat continue to feel the increased extension and width of your back.

Now roll over onto your belly and relax into the mat. Notice your breath and how it contacts the mat. Where are your arms in repose? How are your legs? Turned in or turned out? Or are they each going in opposite directions? Enjoy your breath and abdominal contact with the mat for a few minutes. Let your head move from one side to the other. Do you have a preferred side? Place your hands on the mat beside your shoulders and pressing into the mat send your bum back towards and onto your heels. Leave your hands where they are, allowing your arms and upper back an opening stretch. Encourage the breath into this open back. You will also feel your breath move against your thighs. Send your sit bones towards your heels and little by little your back should release and stretch. Gently open your knees and thighs. Let your belly or your "bowl" relax. This stretch will be felt in the inner leg, right up into the pelvic floor. Don't push this. Explore gently and breathe.

Move up onto all fours à la "doggie" position and wag your tail as if you were pleased to be doing so! Notice the length of your spine from your head to your tail. Relax your belly and breathe. Move your head away from your body and you will find that your body follows. Explore the notion of crawling by leading with the head. Notice how your arms and shoulders extend out of your back. Take yourself for a fundamental crawl about the room, looking up and out. Does the creature in you feel the primary instinct in the movement? Whenever this exercise is done with a student, the cat will watch with great interest as if to say in a disdainful way, "Well, now you are finally teaching movement!" The creature in all of us recognizes the primary instinct in movement. Crawling is the developmental step prior to walking, and reviewing this process allows us to explore the support of the joints and the musculature in movement. Allow your head to lead your body up onto your feet to walk around the room, keeping alive in you the sense of crawling. Can you sense the developmental step forward here?

Spinal Roll

The next step is to learn a simple rolling over, through your spine, touching your toes. Initially people tend to begin this movement by dropping their head forward and down and collapsing the body at the waist, thus cutting the back into segments. In contrast, begin this movement of the spine by tilting the head forward and up. As the diagram indicates, notice how the occipital joint is located where the skull meets the spine; directly behind the uvula (the fleshy extension that hangs down from the middle of the soft palate), inside the centre of the head. You will be looking at your breastbone, as you sense the incremental movement of each vertebra following the head. Do not collapse your shoulders as the chest softens and you lengthen the spine to roll forward. Rather, allow the shoulder girdle to head upwards, towards the ceiling, as you roll. Continue to think of coming up and out of your hips as you extend the "C" curve of the spine. Your large back muscles should be lengthening in the same direction as they follow the direction of your head. Tell your knees and ankles to release or bend a little to counter the feeling of falling forward. Allow your head to hang freely. Release your arms and shoulders. You will feel the greatest amount of stretch in your legs, not in your back. Order your knees to direct away from one another as you play with the flexion and the release of the joints in your legs. This movement should increase the opening of your back and rib cage. The increased width of your back opens more space for breath. As you begin to roll up, continue to maintain flexion in the knees and ankles. Allow your tail bone to gently curl under, initiating an incremental and sequential movement vertebra by vertebra leaving your head to roll up last. Once the head is atop the central axis see out with active eyes. Many people sense their shoulders are too far forward and feel the inclination to adjust them or pull them back. DON'T. Give yourself a moment to observe your balance and the organization of your body – forwardly centred and ready to move.

Connecting Sound to Body

In this standing position, we may begin to release the voice into the breath and the body. Continue to breathe comfortably and with ease. When you experience the impulse (which actors often define as "the need") to begin, allow a gentle hum to connect to the exhalation of your breath. Allow the hum to be short, almost staccato in nature. Do not concern yourself with finding a specific pitch on which to hum. Initially choose a pitch which is easy to find, somewhere in what you feel is the middle of your vocal range. This is an opportunity to find the connection between breath and sound, not to impose the pressure of making a beautiful, professionally trained sound. At this point the feeling of the vibration in the

Figure 5: Alignment of the Body

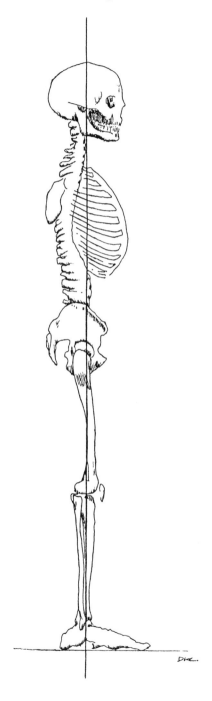

sound is much more important than any auditory feed-back. Therefore, do not judge the quality of your hum. This will inhibit your exploration. <u>Hum with your lips gently touching each other.</u> *If you clench your jaw or press your lips you will inhibit the vibration of the sound from finding its way forward. Initially, do not release sound on every exhalation. Once you relax into the exercise you will find a pattern which seems natural to your own rhythm of breath, remembering that you are a human being and not an automated machine. Most of our problems in travelling from breath on to sound arise out of an unconscious need or desire to control or master the breath, as a means of controlling or mastering our voices. Of course, this effort has exactly the reverse effect. The more we fight our breath the more tension we experience in our voices.*

While doing this exercise observe any tension in your knees. It's manifest in a manner we affectionately call the "locked knee monster:" those people who insist on tightly locking their knees whenever standing still. When our knees are locked most of us hold our breath. In addition, when we stand with our knees tightly locked we have no balance. We are an easy pushover. If we unlock our knees, however, while still maintaining the identical stance, we have much more balance and breath, giving a sense of a greater strength. Many singing teachers insist that if the knees are locked there can be no breath, and without breath there can be no sound. Isn't it interesting then that this locked knee position, which gives us the *feeling* of being strong and balanced, is doing the exact opposite?

Connecting the sound to the body requires a continued heightened physical awareness. Unfortunately, many individuals disregard their newly discovered physical sensations as they begin to incorporate the voice. They seem more concerned with the sound of their voices and forget that their bodies have anything to do with the creation of sound. Therefore, give yourself permission to juggle these two balls at once. There will, no doubt, be moments when you drop one. But a simple reminder enables you to integrate the body and voice as one.

Range

Once the sensation of the sound is gently vibrating on and between your lips we may begin to warm up and open the vocal range. From the initial middle note at which you began to hum, give yourself permission to slowly begin to travel down in pitch. Experiment with how low you can hum without pushing or pressing down; trying find the very bottom of your voice. That is the very lowest note where you can still make sound while feeling its easy vibration on your lips. Perhaps it is lower than you think. If you put your hand on your chest, you will notice while humming in the lower register that you may feel the vibrations of your voice. This sensation has given us the expression "chest voice." As we warm up and open this part of our range it is important to remind ourselves of the principle that we introduced in the physical work: this is a warm-up and not a workout. Therefore, an easy and relaxed breath pattern, accompanied by the gentle vibration of sound on the lips, is of the utmost importance.

When you feel comfortable with humming the lower pitches, continue travelling up towards the middle of your range and beyond. As you hum upwards you will sense a change in the placement; the strong sensation that you experienced in your chest will subside as you grow increasingly aware of the inside of your mouth and the very small sinus cavities in your head. This placement of the resonance has come to be known as the "head voice." As we hum higher pitches we experience a change in our sensory feedback. For example, higher pitches may feel smaller or weaker when compared to the feeling experienced in the chest voice. However, encourage your breath pattern to be easy. At higher pitches, increased tension in the breath may initiate both a locking of the jaw and a tightening of the neck muscles that will inevitably stop the vibration of the vocal folds. Therefore, self-awareness is crucial in warming up and opening this part of your vocal range. In contrast to tension, offer the direction to soften and relax, thereby encouraging a more easy breath. This ex-

ploration encourages the upper notes in your voice to be free. As you did with the the exploration of the chest voice, give yourself the opportunity to play and explore in the head voice. Remember that the map is not necessarily the territory. If your habitual vocal use limits you to speaking in the bottom of your voice these pitches will seem strange at first. But persevere.

After you are comfortable with these pitches, allow yourself to integrate these two extreme ends of your vocal range by sliding gently up and down while you hum; connecting the head and chest voice together in a seemingly smooth and seamless manner. At first you may experience a shift in the voice as you glide back and forth between the head and the chest – many voice teachers refer to this change as "the break." Through the experience of the gentle hum we facilitate a connection through this break, thereby providing people with opportunities to use more of their natural voice.

Focusing the Voice

Now that your voice is warm and vibrant throughout the fullness of its range we may begin to release this sound into the space around us. Mindful of the ease in our bodies and breath, begin each line of the following exercise with a hum, gently vibrating between the lips, then releasing it onto the voice through the following sequence:

EE as in the word 'leaf'

AY as in the word 'lace'

AH as in the word 'lost'

OH as in the word 'load'

OO as in the word 'lose'

Then try:

BEE	**BAY**	**BAH**	**BOH**	**BOO**
MEE	**MAY**	**MAH**	**MOH**	**MOO**
DEE	**DAY**	**DAH**	**DOH**	**DOO**

SEE	*SAY*	*SAH*	*SOH*	*SOO*
LEE	*LAY*	*LAH*	*LOH*	*LOO*
KEE	*KAY*	*KAH*	*KOH*	*KOO*

Do not initiate speech with a whisper or breathy quality to the sound. This is referred to as "de-voicing" and does not engage the breath or the vocal folds in the manner required for full and healthy communication. Do not lose the vibration of the hum as you drop your jaw and come onto sound. This transition also must feel seamless. Releasing the hum through sound into the space around your body is a natural progression from releasing the hum into the space inside your body. Focus your sound into the room, directing it towards a focal point as you remain centred.

Check in with your body, your breath, the ease of the connection onto the voice, and feel the openness of the "vocal channel" from the bottom of your "bowl" up and out into the world around you.

Speech and Language

The final, but most important, step in the warm up is to release this free and open voice into words. This progression may be accomplished through the use of simple tongue twisters and eventually, to a piece of text such as a sonnet or song. Our articulators (the lips, teeth, tongue and soft palate) play an integral part in opening and maintaining the freedom of the voice.

For many speakers the following exercise demonstrates that during daily vocal use, the engagement of their articulators is minimal. Therefore, through this part of the warm-up you may sense that you are developing a manner of speech which is foreign and perhaps, insincere. The point, however, is not to adopt an exaggerated accent as a result of engaging our articulators, but rather to find a clear and specific use of the articulators which will support our voices.

Begin slowly and carefully, remembering not to push. Feel the light but very specific contact of the articulators through each word. Allow the openness that you have discovered in the voice to continue. Do not inhibit your voice as you begin to work on articulation.

Tongue Twisters:

1. A pale pink proud peacock pompously preened its pretty plumage.
2. A blue-backed blackbird blew big bubbles.
3. A tidy tiger tied a tie tighter to tidy her tiny tail.
4. Vera valued the valley violets.
5. Maggie MacGregor makes magnificent macaroons.
6. Whether the weather be fine
   Or whether the weather be not,
   Whether the weather be cold
   Or whether the weather be hot,
   We'll weather the weather
   Whatever the weather,
   Whether we like it or not. (Parkin, 1969)
7. Cameron Campbell is a crazy, crooked critic from Calgary. (Pearson)

The final step is to connect this open and supported voice with a sonnet or a song. If this suggestion does not meet the demands which you encounter as professional teachers, you may want to find a more appropriate text. The sonnet or song is merely a tool providing an opportunity to connect your voice to language. Once this connection has been experienced and reinforced, it is not limited to text but becomes available to all possibilities of communication.

Give yourself the opportunity to breathe, to speak slowly and to articulate and taste each word. Our connection to language is often the most difficult as we are reluctant to give ourselves the time to explore and experience the richness. Remind yourself that this text is not a grocery list and deserves your full-bodied attention.

As an unperfect actor on the stage,
Who with his fear is put besides his part,
Or some fierce thing replete with too much rage,

Whose strength's abundance weakens his own heart;
So I, for fear of trust, forget to say
The perfect ceremony of love's rite,
And in mine own love's strength seem to decay,
O'ercharged with burden of mine own love's might.
O, let my books be then the eloquence
And dumb presagers of my speaking breast,
Who plead for love and look for recompense
More than that tongue that more hath more expressed.
O, learn to read what silent love hath writ;
To hear with eyes belongs to love's fine wit.

(Shakespeare, "Sonnet 23")

Conclusion – Janine Pearson

The work presented in this chapter provides opportunities to explore our full potential as efficient and effective speakers. This communication begins with the breath and the body, and eventually releases itself onto sound and into language. The exercises we have shared are meant to be accessible and practical in their application; they serve to demystify this process. Learning about one's voice is not an academic exercise, but a full-bodied experience. To learn about one's voice is to gain a greater understanding of one's body and breath. Therefore, in the journey to discover our voices we inevitably discover ourselves. Teachers who speak from a position of self-discovery will undoubtedly assist their students to do the same.

Recommended References

Voice Books

Berry, Cicely. *The Actor and His Text.* London: Harrap, 1988.

Berry, Cicely. *Your Voice and How to Use it Successfully.* London: Harrap, 1987.

Boone, Daniel R. *Is Your Voice Telling On You? How to Find Your Natural Voice.* San Diego, CA: Singular Publishing Group, 1991.

Bunch, Meribeth. *Dynamics of the Singing Voice.* New York: Springer-Verlag, 1993.

Linklater, Kristin. *Freeing the Natural Voice.* New York: Drama Book Specialists, 1976.

McCallion, Michael. *The Voice Book*. London: Faber and Faber, 1988.

Miller, Richard. *The Structure of Singing: System and Art in Vocal Technique*. New York: Schrimer Books, 1986.

Rodenburg, Patsy. *The Right to Speak*. London: Methuen Drama, 1992.

Rodenburg, Patsy. *The Need for Words*. London: Methuen Drama, 1993.

Alexander Books

Alexander, F. Matthias. *The Use of the Self*. Downey, CA: Centerline Press, 1984.

Gelb, Michael. *Body Learning: An Introduction to the Alexander Technique*. New York: Henry Holt and Company, 1981.

Leibowitz, Judy and Connington, Bill. *The Alexander Technique*. New York: Harper Collins Publishers, 1991.

Other

Parkin, Ken. *Anthology of British Tongue Twisters*. London: Samuel French, 1969.

Pearson, Janine. Unpublished Documents. August 10, 1993.

Shakespeare, William. "Sonnet 23." Ed. T.J.B. Spencer. *The Sonnets and A Lover's Complaint*. London: Penguin, 1988, p. 88.

Certified Teachers of the Alexander Technique

*For information and a comprehensive list of teachers
in these countries write to the following:*

Canada:

Canadian Society of Teachers of the Alexander Technique

P. O. Box 47025, #19 - 555 W. 12th Ave.,

Vancouver, British Columbia. V5Z 3X0

United States:

North American Society of Teachers of the Alexander
Technique

P. O. Box 5536,

Playa del Rey, California. 90296

United Kingdom and Other Countries:

Society of Teachers of the Alexander Technique

10 London House

266 Fulham Road,

London, England. SW10 9EL

JANINE PEARSON is a voice coach with the Stratford Shakespeare Theatre in Stratford, Ontario, and Head of Voice at the National Theatre School of Canada, Montreal. She has worked in theatres and universities across Canada, in the U.S.A. and in Britain. In addition, she teaches and coaches singers, broadcasters, executives and teachers. In 1991, she founded, in conjunction with the Education Department at the Stratford Festival, "Voice Care and Development Workshops for Teachers." She holds an Advanced Diploma in Voice Studies from the Central School of Speech and Drama in London, England; has pursued singing and languages studies at the Humboldt Institut in Ratzenried, Germany; and has a B. Music in singing and a B.F.A. in acting from the University of Regina, Saskatchewn.

KELLY MCEVENUE graduated from the American Center for the Alexander Tehnique in 1980. She is the Alexander Technique Coach for the Stratford Shakespeare Festival in Stratford, Ontario. In addition, she is a member of the faculty at Ryerson Theatre School, Toronto, and the University of Toronto Opera School. She has taught at the Guildhall School of Music and Drama and the Centre for the Development and Graduate Training in the Alexander Teachnique, London, England. She has also coached at the Shaw Festival and the Citadel Theatre. In 1992, she began teaching collaboratively with Janine Pearson on "Voice Care and Development for Teachers." Ms. McEvenue has taught movement in several voice-intensive workshops with Patsy Rodenburg, with Equity Showcase Theatre, Toronto, and the Royal National Theatre, London, England.

DAVID ROSS is a visual artist who lives in Stratford, Ontario, where he works for the Festival. He did the illustrations in this chapter.

CHAPTER 4

Preventing and Reducing Pathology

Alanna McDonough and Elizabeth Hunt

As Speech Pathologists who specialize in voice therapy, a large percentage of our clients are professional voice users. Teachers and coaches make up a substantial part of the professional voice user group. This chapter was written with teachers and coaches in mind to provide them with information about how the voice works, what prevents the voice from working and, finally, how to prevent and treat the disordered voice.

How the Voice Works

Our voices are the result of a balance between the basic mechanisms of breathing, phonation (vocal cord vibration) and resonance. The primary purpose of these systems is to assist in life support; however, they have also evolved to operate the process of voice production. While it is convenient to discuss these three systems separately, it is important to remember that they are highly interdependent for the production of voice.

1. Respiratory System

The respiratory tract can be divided into two parts, the upper and the lower. The upper respiratory tract is composed of the nasal cavity, oral cavity, pharynx and the larynx. The lower respiratory tract is composed of the trachea, the two bronchi and the lungs (Figure 1).

The course of the upper respiratory tract is F-shaped. For people who breathe through the uppermost entrance, air passes through the nose to the nasopharynx and from there through a muscular valve, called the velopharyngeal port. For

Figure 1: Respiratory System

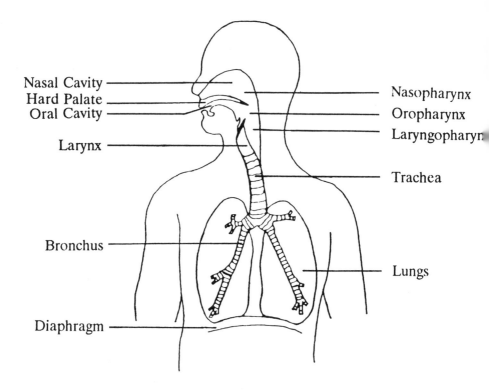

individuals who breathe through the lower entrance, air flow is through the mouth, oral cavity and into the oropharynx. The air then continues to move through the laryngopharynx and down into the larynx. After the larynx, it passes between the vocal cords, and downward into the trachea. The trachea divides into two branches and into two bronchi that enter the lungs. Below the lungs the diaphragm, the primary muscle of inhalation, separates the chest and the abdomen. As we breathe in, the chest and the lungs expand because of chest muscle contractions and the downward movement of the diaphragm. When the chest muscles and the diaphragm relax, the chest and the lungs become smaller. This decrease in the size of the lungs increases air pressure within them, thus air is exhaled. An analogy of this process is the rib cage expanding, drawing air in like bellows, and as the air is exhaled the muscles relax like a floating parachute.

Respiration or breathing is often referred to as the "fuel" that powers the voice. The three types of breathing we do differs depending upon the activity. Simply stated, these are silent breathing (i.e., sleeping, sitting, watching TV, etc.), speech breathing and exercise breathing (i.e., rapid panting or long distance running). Silent breathing has a more regular in and out cycle of air. Speech breathing involves a more rapid inhalation of air and then a slow exhalation of air during which speech is produced. As the air is exhaled, it passes through the vocal cords sending them into vibration, which gives us voice.

Since air is the fuel that runs our voice, it is important when we are speaking take time to regularly replenish our air. This goal is accomplished by pausing during speaking. As we pause, our chest expands again, we take in a new breath and we continue talking. The breathing cycle happens automatically during pause time. However, an ineffective speech-breathing sequence can be changed: inhalations can be made more efficient and exhalations controlled. Both the quality and loudness of our voice are affected by our breathing cycle. Generally a loud, strong voice requires more air than a whispered, breathy voice. Overall, effective speech breathing should be done in a rhythmical, relaxed manner.

Figure 2: Looking Down at the Vocal Cords

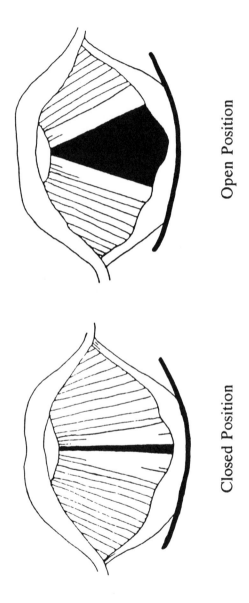

Open Position

Closed Position

2. Phonatory System

While the production of voice is dependent upon all three systems (respiratory, phonatory and resonatory), the system that actually produces voice is the phonatory system. It consists of the larynx and all of the muscles and ligaments that hold it together and move its parts. The larynx serves as a valve entranceway to the lower respiratory tract. Its most important biological role is that of an airway protector to prevent food or liquids from entering the lungs during swallowing. With regard to voice, all incoming and outgoing lung air must pass through the valve-like vocal cords. If the vocal cords are open, the air simply passes through and is exhaled (see Figure 2). However, if voice is required, the vocal cords are brought together and the exhaled air sends them into vibration producing voice. How tightly or loosely the vocal cords are brought together affects the quality of the voice. A breathy voices results from vocal cords that do not come together fully or are kept open in a strained manner. On the other hand, vocal cords squeeze too firmly together result in a harsh, strained vocal quality.

The size of our vocal cords also changes the pitch of our voice. For example, women's vocal cords tend to be shorter and thinner; thus, faster vibrations result in a higher pitched voice. Male vocal cords, which tend to be longer and thicker, vibrate more slowly and result in a lower pitch. Here the analogy of a stringed instrument may be beneficial. A violin has different string thicknesses. The size of the string, tension of the string and the force exerted by the bow result in various pitches.

3. Resonatory System

Resonance plays an important role in the amplification and projection of our voices. This vocal concept is illustrated well if we think of the strength and tone of an opera singer, who because of technique, generates the type of sound which can be heard over a full orchestra.

The resonatory, or amplifier, system is made up of cavities situated above the vocal cords: the throat, mouth, and the nose. The primary source of resonance is the throat (pharynx). The walls of the throat are made up of sphincter muscles

Figure 3: Resonatory System

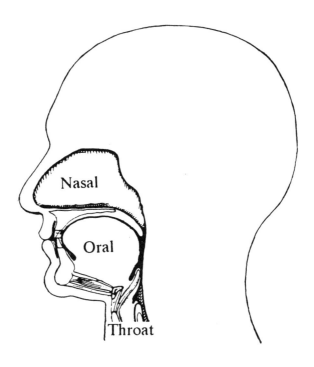

which contract and relax becoming larger or smaller depending on the level of tension. Additional areas of resonance include the oral cavity and the nasal cavity (see Figure 3).

A voice with the most ideal resonance and tone appears to result from a open, relaxed throat that allows air being exhaled to move through in the throat, oral and nasal areas. In addition to tense or relaxed throat muscles, tongue placement and tongue tension in the oral area affects where the air vibrates. For example a tongue pushed far back in the mouth blocks optimal air flow to the oral and nasal cavities, causing damping of sound.

A healthy, effective voice results from the coordination and effective use of the three systems: respiration, phonation and resonation. Problems in any one of these areas can limit the professional voice user and possibly develop into a voice disorder. Voice disorders are commonly divided into organic and non-organic. Organic disorders are those during which the patient suffers a "physical condition" (i.e., neurological impairment resulting from a stroke). The disability also may be congenital or one which develops over time. Non-organic disorders are those that do not begin as physical in nature, but which may develop into an organic problem (i.e., vocal cord nodules).

These non-organic disorders may develop when excessive muscular contraction and force of movement in one or more of the previously mentioned systems occurs. Ineffective and inappropriate muscle use is referred to as "vocal hyperfunction." While not all voice disorders are the result of vocal hyperfunction, for the purposes of this chapter, voice disorders resulting from hyperfunction are the focus.

What Prevents the Voice from Working

1. Vocal Hyperfunction

Vocal hyperfunction is discussed with reference to the three previously described systems: respiration, phonation and resonation.

Hyperfunction of the respiratory system occurs in people with normal voices as well as among voice-disordered persons. The primary difference is that people who do not suffer a voice disorder tolerate hyperfunctional breathing while the voice-disordered individual cannot tolerate these breathing inefficiencies.

Respiration problems can occur during either the inhalation or exhalation phase of breathing. Often the amount of air inhaled is not sufficient for what the individual attempts to say on that breath. Another difficulty occurs when the inhalation has been sufficient, but the speaker attempts to speak beyond his/her inhalation limits (i.e., saying too many words per breath) or speaks beyond a comfortable breath phrase. Taking too much air on inhalation can also present difficulties during controlled exhalation. Another difficulty occurs among speakers who let out too much air early in their verbalization so that by the time they have reached the end, they are out of breath. Most normal speakers appear to closely match the prolonged timing of their exhalation to the length of verbalization they wish to say. Patients with vocal hyperfunction often do not demonstrate a normal exhalation that matches spoken verbalization. They show signs of effort and struggle with breathing when they attempt to voice results. Examples of problems include shallow clavicular breathing, tight throat or abdominal muscles, and holding the breath.

Hyperfunction of the phonatory system is most often noted on the vocal cords which are covered by a membrane very sensitive to irritation. Irritation to this area results from simply using too much effort, tension or pressure when speaking so that the vocal cords come together too tightly or the entire laryngeal area is squeezed or pressed. The individual who uses an inappropriate pitch level irritates the vocal cords. Whether too high or too low a pitch, unnecessary muscle energy is required because the vocal cords adjust in length and mass to produce the artificial voice. The individual who speaks with unnecessary precision, who often sounds as if he or she is "punching out" the beginning and end of each and every word often has an hyperfunctional problem. Referred to as a hard glottal attack, over a period of time this problem leads to vocal cord irritation.

Hyperfunction of the resonatory system is primarily related to muscle tension or articulator positioning that does not allow the air to move through the throat, oral and nasal resonating areas. With a normal voice, vocal cord vibrations created by air flowing through them produce a sound that then is amplified by the resonating areas of the vocal tract. Changes to this vocal tract such as tight throat muscles, tongue positions in the oral cavity, a rigid, clenched jaw or blocked/swollen tissues from cold or allergies adversely affect the resonance of the voice because of ineffective vibrations in the throat, oral or nasal cavities.

If the three voice-production systems do not interact effectively, the resulting voice will often need remedial voice therapy. In addition to vocal production problems, external influences also lead to voice difficulties. These external influences, including "vocal hygiene" and the abuse or misuse of the voice, are discussed in the following section.

Aspects of Vocal Dysfunction

In addition to the physical production systems within the body that may contribute to vocal dysfunction, a number of external influences can contribute to vocal disabilities. Behavioral, physiological and environmental influences must be considered when assessing how the voice functions in an efficient and effective manner.

In each area, because of professional demands, teachers have particular difficulties, while coaches often have similar problems.

1. Behavioral Influences

Day to day behaviors and habits influence our voices tremendously. Understanding daily vocal demands, vocal habits, postures and lifestyle, and the advantages of voice training will provide a better use and health of the voice.

With regard to vocal demand, teachers are required to speak for long periods of time without breaks and often under stress. They use different voices to inspire, control, excite, provoke and console. Teachers speak over background noise, in large open spaces, or over the loud sounds of singing or cheering voices. Each one of these daily activities places excess demand on the voice. In addition, teachers may have active vocal lives outside of the classroom. The teacher whose voice suffers from classroom fatigue goes home to do more talking.

Excessive and demanding voice use requires better than average vocal behaviors. A teacher must learn to vary the amount of continuous talking time and to take short vocal breaks. Using tools such as whistles and gestures to gain attention rather than using the voice will save unnecessary fatigue. Vocal habits affect the systems that produce the voice. Loudness, speaking pitch, voice quality and breathing patterns are subject to misuse through bad habits. Teachers need to vary loudness according to the circumstances. Moving closer to the listener reduces the demand for increasing loudness. Responding to signs of vocal fatigue is absolutely necessary in maintaining vocal health.

Vocal role models, culture and personal expectations all influence our vocal habits. Like most habits we learn behaviors unwittingly and are often unaware of the negative impact. Understanding personal vocal habits will help teachers correct damaging behaviors. For example, many teachers have been told by their spouses or children to "turn off the 'teacher' voice." Getting the listener's attention before starting to speak will also preserve the voice. Teachers are often guilty of using their voice to get attention, continuing to talk when they aren't being heard, or using their "teacher" voice even when it's not necessary.

Primary or singing teachers often use a high pitched voice to match or model the children. Inappropriate and prolonged use of a too high a pitch will cause fatigue and potential vocal damage.

A rough, gravelly voice is often the consequence of voice fatigue or lack of warm-up (early morning voice). It can also be the result of bad habits or an imitation of other voice models. In some instances a person may continue to use a rough, gravelly or hoarse voice after developing a bad habit during a bout of laryngitis. If the voice continues to be dysphonic after the infection has cleared up, then the speaker has developed a habit that must be corrected because habitual behaviors ultimately cause a physical change in the larynx. It is remarkable how quickly poor vocal habits are learned.

Most teachers have an adequate air supply for speaking, but commonly they use poor breathing habits that tax the sound system. A poor breather will take inefficient breaths, work while getting air into the lung, speak well past the comfortable breath phrase, or maintain poor posture making breathing difficult. Taking shallow breaths by lifting the rib cage (and shoulders) results in the need to replenish more often. Making a noise while grabbing or gulping in air is inefficient and damaging. Squeezing out the last bit of air while speaking is tiring and creates a need to gasp for more breath. Breathing should be relaxed and effortless. Learning to pay attention to good breathing behaviors will greatly assist the speaker.

An interesting phenomenon occurs when a speaker increases the speaking rate (speed). Although there is no direct link between the speed one speaks and the pitch or loudness, fast speakers often use louder and higher-pitched voices than they normally use. In addition, they shift to shallow breathing patterns, thus creating a strain on the voice.

Yelling, cheering, excessive coughing, throat clearing, pushing or forcing sound from the throat are all considered abusive behaviors. Many speakers force or pop the vocal cords together (hard glottal attack) to accentuate a point or get attention. Forceful use of the vocal cords causes the laryngeal muscles to become fatigued and alters the delicate mucous lining of the vocal cords. This type of vocal assault will likely result in increased mucous production that sets up a continuous need to clear the throat. These habits are largely avoidable and can be exchanged for less damaging behaviors.

The voice is very much a part of the entire body. Posture, head/neck and shoulder positioning, muscle tension and jaw opening (to name a few) influence the voice we produce. Understanding the entire body and its relationship to sound production is vital in producing and maintaining a good voice. In addition, the general state of health, diet, stress management, and habits including alcohol, caffeine consumption, as well as smoking and drug use are lifestyle issues that affect the voice. Alcohol, caffeine, smoke and many prescription and non-prescription drugs are damaging: most are particularly drying to the throat and contribute to vocal disability.

Racing car drivers understand how the automobile works before getting behind the wheel of a car. They also understand the need to train for long periods to increase physical strength and fast reflexes to improve their ability to respond to demanding situations. Yet, most teachers who are "vocal racing drivers" in the classroom rarely have a single lesson in how the voice works or what they must do to protect such an essential skill. Teachers would benefit from learning how the voice works, what prevents it from working properly, and how to develop a regular vocal fitness program to prevent voice problems from occurring.

2. Physiological Influences

Although physical makeup may be determined at birth, other physiological changes can influence the voice. The general state of health, accidents, injuries, surgical procedures, hormonal changes, medications, fitness and diet, emotional/psychological status, fatigue and humidification are among the influences that affect the way we sound.

Although no one controls the fact that emergent health issues may negatively affect the voice, anyone can make certain that the influence of these factors is kept under control or that every other negative vocal influence is managed with vigilance. For instance, someone with exercise-induced asthma cannot behave as others do and must accept this limitation.

Teachers with a history of asthma, bronchitis, allergies, frequent upper respiratory infections or stomach problems will have added burdens in the professional voice arena. These people will have to take precautions to avoid stimuli which aggravate the problem. They have to be better than average in caring and maintaining the voice as well as their overall health. They may be required to do physical exercises or to do voice warm-ups on a regular basis, thus reducing the impact of the underlying physiological conditions.

A note of caution is necessary. Asthmatic patients take medication to combat frightening and dangerous symptoms related to breathing, but it must be understood that many of the inhalants alter the laryngeal tissues. Many non-prescription drugs also cause dryness. Bronchitis may result in habitual coughing, and asthma sufferers may use a shallow upper chest breathing pattern. Many over-the-counter and prescription medications have a negative influence on the voice. Aspirin, antihistamines, diuretics and some medications used in patients with hypertension and heart disease may cause changes in voice quality or production.

Gastro-esophageal reflex (GER) can have a significant impact on the voice. Until recently people with voice disorders were unaware that they had GER, and of the influence it had on the voice. There are a host of symptoms which may be present in people with GER. The most common are a tickling or burning sensation in the throat or feeling of a lump in the throat, a bitter taste, regurgitation, frequent burping, morning or chronic hoarseness, and heartburn. A diagnosis can be made through a testing procedure or, more commonly, through a trial period of behavior modification such as raising the head of the bed, altering the diet, and taking prescribed medication.

Many other general health conditions that affect the respiratory system and musculoskeletal systems may influence vocal function. Among these are temporomandibular disorders (TMD), hormonal influences, injuries, accidents and surgery.

Temporomandibular Disorders may be caused by bad habits, stress, injury or other physiological factors. The syndrome is a condition affecting the mouth opening which is extremely important in voice production. While there are many symptoms related to TMD, the most common in patients with voice disorders include restricted or painful jaw opening, clenching or grinding teeth, sore tongue and throat, laryngitis, stiffness or pain in the neck or face, frequent coughing or throat clearing, and difficulty swallowing. Proper assessment and treatment by a dentist are necessary.

The hormonal system is a highly sensitive system that has a significant effect on the human voice. Hormone changes may result in an alteration of the fluid content of the laryngeal muscles, thus affecting the shape and size of the muscles. Hormonal disorders such as hypothyroidism or pancreatic dysfunction can cause vocal change. The most dramatic hormonal change occurs in adolescent boys and girls during puberty. Adult voices also are affected by hormonal changes. For instance, the hormonal impact in menstruating (approximately 50% of the population), pregnant or postmenopausal women may cause changes such as more limited vocal range, voice fatigue, slight hoarseness or poor voice quality. Medications used to treat hormone-related problems may cause the voice to become unsteady or lower the vocal pitch; some vocal changes resulting from hormonal alterations or pharmacological treatment are permanent.

Vocal injury and/or surgery should forewarn a speaker that he or she is vulnerable to vocal disability. Laryngeal surgery requires the alteration of a very delicate muscle and mucosal lining. Even with the advancement of surgical techniques such as laser technology, the vocal cords are vulnerable to permanent alteration in how they produce sound. Other surgical procedures of any bodily system relating to vocal production will influence the voice. Spinal, neck, shoulder or jaw injury or surgery may affect the voice. Muscle injury causing a change in physical behavior potentially impacts the voice. In addition, many surgical procedures require intubation, a procedure which frequently irritates the vocal cords.

Poor diet and lack of exercise result in poor overall health. A healthy voice results from a healthy, well-nourished, rested body. Adequate moisture level in the body is crucial for a healthy voice. The amount of fluid intake as well as the environmental humidity conditions cannot be overemphasized in maintaining vocal health. Humidifiers, steaming and increasing liquid (non-caffeine) help combat dryness.

As well, the voice is an excellent indicator of emotional status. Teachers who are under stress or who suffer from psychological and emotional problems will often demonstrate voice differences. Emotional states such as anxiety and depression are particularly noticeable in the voice. These conditions have psychological, physical and vocal manifestations. It is always important to treat the underlying cause of the psychological disturbance; it may also be necessary to treat the vocal symptoms.

3. Environmental Influences

Speaking voices are greatly influenced by the environment in which they are asked to perform. Environmental factors not only influence the way we produce sound, but the way we react. We tend to become more loud in large or noisy environments.

Teachers need also to assess the acoustics of the schools in which they work from the perspective of voice care. Room size and distances between speaker and listeners should also be considered. Large cavernous spaces that reflect sound cause a speaker to shout or to compensate for lack of feedback. When speaking in noisy outside environments, teachers often push their voices to be heard and to combat the feeling that sound is being lost. Considering the effects of the acoustics, and the reaction to them helps prevent unnecessary vocal effort.

Speaking over classroom noise, in the gymnasium, or in competition with other sounds or voices often results in increased vocal effort. Large audiences create more noise and require louder voices to be heard as well as to keep attention. Competing noises such as fans, street noises, students shuffling or engine (car) noises need to be considered when talking. Speakers need to use the voice efficiently and without abusive behaviors in such environments.

In addition to noisy environments, the physical plant and the climate may create environments that irritate teachers' voices. Older schools may be environmentally unfit because high levels of dust, mites and fungus may be present. New schools, on the other hand, may have sealed windows reducing exposure to fresh air. Forced air heating and cooling systems can be equally drying to the throat. Strong solvents and disinfectants are used in schools to maintain high levels of hygiene; however, these solutions often irritate the voice. Smoke, fumes and pollution are natural enemies of the voice. Many people are allergic to these common everyday irritants, some of which are located in staff rooms. The Canadian winter is a harsh climate for voices. Long periods of time spent outside breathing in dry cold air will be detrimental. The average Canadian adult has at least two colds a year; school age children catch anywhere from six to twelve. During the school year, teachers often work in close contact with an entire roomful of sneezing and coughing children. For most, a common cold or flu usually represents nothing more than a temporary setback. Nevertheless, for teachers, the local fallout from these mild illnesses could be cause for concern. More than most professionals, teachers are likely to be exposed to illnesses that may influence vocal health. Becoming aware of vulnerability to illness requires vigilance in maintaining good health. Some of these conditions are, of course, a "normal" condition of living in Canada, but because of the need to speak so much, teachers need to be aware of these constraints and perhaps educate others about potential vocal problems.

Preventing & Treating Voice Disorders

The human voice is an efficient and hearty mechanism that continues to work throughout an entire life. It can withstand numerous assaults and traumas and generally recovers fully. However there are limits to the abuse it can receive and it will eventually breakdown if not maintained properly. Prevention of voice disorders is the first line of defense for teachers. A clear understanding of how the voice works, what will have a negative impact on the voice and when to practice vocal hygiene and proper voice use prevents most voice disorders from occurring.

Remediation of a voice disorder is hard work and requires a more vigilant approach to achieve full recovery of a healthy voice. A teacher diagnosed with a voice disorder will have learned about voice use and voice health, and will have been taught corrective exercises and techniques for proper voice technique. Compensatory strategies, such as amplification or non-verbal communication such as writing or hand signals, may have to be incorporated into the classroom. Health, psychological and emotional, and behavioral issues must be addressed. A teacher who has suffered a vocal injury or who has chronic voice problems such as voice loss or hoarseness every September, requires a thorough evaluation, diagnosis and treatment. Teachers who have recovered the use of their voice need to continue practicing good vocal behavior.

1. Voice Evaluation:

Evaluation of a voice can involve a number of participants. A collaborative approach is the best way to assess the patient with a voice disorder. In addition to self-assessment, teachers with voice concerns could obtain support from family, colleagues and students. Voice care professionals include otolaryngologists (ENT doctors), speech and language pathologists, voice therapists, vocal coaches and singing teachers, and a variety of medical specialists including allergists, goastroenterologists and dentists to name a few. Keeping a vocal diary is an important part of voice change. A teacher needs to have an accurate record of the amount of time spent talking, under what conditions and to what effect. Then, a teacher may begin to notice patterns that will help in changing behaviors.

The teacher must first learn to listen to his/her own voice. Using a tape recorder or listening to answering machine or voice mail message provides feedback and permits objectivity if the message isn't interpreted subjectively. Hearing the voice and detecting bad habits is the first step in changing behaviors.

Colleagues and spouses may be able to give feedback about vocal habits. However, be careful about whom is asked to be "vocal police." A teacher may be more sensitive about the voice than she or he realizes and this request could definitely strain relationships. Students are often eager to learn about their bodies and willing to assist if they know about a problem.

During a medical examinations, an otolaryngologist (ENT doctor) constructs a visual image of the vocal cords to determine the condition of the structure and function of the vocal cords. It is important to know if the vocal cords are infected or if there is any alteration in the size or shape of the cords. Irregular movement or paralysis will be detected by the ENT doctor. The ENT exam may include videostroboscopy which provides the examiner and patient with valuable information about how the cords are functioning. This instrument can also be used as a biofeedback tool in retraining voice use.

Based on the findings during the ENT examination other medical referrals may be indicated. A therapeutic program may include referrals to other services to assist in stress management, lifestyle changes, diet alteration and exercise/relaxation programs. It may also include consultation and referral to voice professionals such as vocal coaches, singing coaches or Alexander teachers, to name a few. Allergists, respirologists, psychiatrists, physiotherapists, dietitians and speech and language pathologists are among those medical specialists that may be consulted if remedial vocal care is necessary. A therapy or re-training program may include lifestyle changes, diet alteration, exercise routines, vocal hygiene programs and voice exercises.

The speech language pathologist (SLP) will use auditory, perceptual, physiological and acoustic means to assess the voice output. In addition the SLP will require a detailed case history to properly assess the various influences affecting the voice. Physical condition, respiration, articulation, pitch, loudness, resonance and quality are assessed. Patients are assessed both in terms of what they do habitually as well as what they are capable of doing. The speech/language pathologist attempts to identify all contributing factors and their relative influence on vocal function. As a result of a thorough evaluation, an extensive case history and medical reports, a plan of action is devised. Most voice disorders are not simple or caused by one behavior or condition. An effective treatment/re-training program to improve vocal function will likely require a broad range of activities.

Voice therapy includes an explanation of the problem, identification of vocal abuse & misuse of the voice (see the Vocal Hygiene Table at the end of this chapter) and voice exercises. Voice exercises will address each of the systems that influence the voice: physical, respiratory, phonatory, resonatory and articulatory.

Physical exercises to improve posture and movement will be taught. These exercises may be enhanced by having the patient take other instruction in yoga or the Alexander method. Facial, tongue and jaw exercises are used to increase awareness of tension, improve flexibility and increase articulatory precision. Relaxation exercises may also be taught.

With regard to respiration, patients generally have an adequate air supply, but they use it incorrectly. Exercises to increase awareness of how to breathe and how to manage the breath supply are taught. The most common breathing problems include inefficient inhalation (using the upper chest) or infrequent intake of air (speaking too long without taking a breath in). Some patients lose a lot of air by using a breathy voice or by forcing out too much air when they speak. The voice user must learn to get air in and out of the lungs efficiently and without effort.

Phonation exercises primarily address pitch and vocal effort. To improve the speaking quality of the voice, patients are taught about phonation, pitch, resonance and articulation. The patient learns to identify and develop a habitual speaking voice throughout a comfortable and natural speaking pitch range. Exercises to increase the vocal range may also be taught. Exercises to identify and reduce unnecessary laryngeal force and effort are necessary to maintain or develop the quality of the voice.

Resonance exercises assist in improving teachers' projection. Teachers may learn to increase the power of their voices or change the way in which they produce sound so that it cuts through the noise. An example of this approach would be to use a nasal "twang." Exercises to improve a balance between oral (mouth) and nasal (nose) resonance are taught. Speakers will also learn to take advantage of the oral-pharyngeal cavity (back of the throat) to improve voice quality and amplification. Improving articulation precision and clarity often helps to improve audibility. Clear speech compensates for lack of vocal power: words said clearly may be spoken softly. Exercises to increase tongue mobility as well as jaw opening exercises assist the voice patient to pronounce consonants and say vowels more precisely.

The speech and language pathologist works as a coach and director providing the most efficient and comprehensive road to recovery, but the teacher has the greater challenge: changing habits that have been very firmly established. It is a tremendous challenge to incorporate these new behaviors into every speaking activity. Although it's a cumbersome task, the result is promising. If teacher-voice patients eliminate vocal abuses, develop more effective vocal patterns and address other physiological/behavioral issues, they have an excellent chance for full recovery. Teachers and coaches who become voice patients have a powerful motivation for improving vocal habits: their professional lives depend upon their ability to learn better vocal habits, to develop strategies that reduce abuse and to maintain their voices.

Vocal Hygiene Practice

Avoid Vocal Abuse such as:

Throat clearing.

Yelling, screaming, shouting.

Coughing and vocal sneezing.

Competing with loud noises.

Speaking for long periods without vocal breaks.

Speaking to large groups without amplification.

Speaking or singing with a tired or sore throat.

Singing in the wrong pitch range.

Making vocal noises.

Laughing in a forced voice.

Avoid Vocal Misuse such as:

Whispering.

Using a breathy/protected voice.

Using a habitually loud voice.

Using hard glottal attack.

Speaking in a rough/gravelly voice.

Speaking with a forced voice.

Speaking in the wrong pitch range.

Speaking without proper air supply.

Speaking with tense body/facial muscles.

Speaking with a small mouth opening.

Speaking with poor or imprecise articulation.

Practise Vocal Health Habits such as:

Stretching & relaxation exercises.

Warming-up the voice before speaking.

Watching your posture.

Keeping neck, shoulders & jaw free of tension.

Increasing vocal capabilities through voice exercise.

Increasing the number of "vocal breaks" taken.

Increasing humidity at work and home.

Drinking more water.

Drinking warm liquids after exposure to cold.

Covering your mouth in cold weather.

Avoiding smoking.

Limiting caffeine & alcohol.

Maintaining excellent health.

Recommended Readings

Boone, D. *The Voice and Voice Therapy*, Englewood Cliffs, NJ: Prentice-Hall, 1983.

Boone, D. *Is Your Voice Telling On You?* San Diego, CA: Singular Publishing Group Inc., 1991.

Greene, M. and Mathieson, L. *The Voice and its Disorders,* London: Whurr Publishers, 1989.

Miller, R. *The Structure of Singing*, New York: Schirmer Books, Collier MacMillan Publishers, 1986.

Morrison, M. and Rammage, L. *The Management of Voice Disorders*, San Diego, CA: Singular Publishing Group Inc., 1994.

Prater, R. and Swift, R. *Manual of Voice Therapy*, Boston: Little, Brown and Company, 1984.

Sataloff, R.T. *Professional Voice: The Science and Art of Clinical Care*, New York: Raven Press Ltd., 1991.

Sies, L. *Voice and Voice Disorders*. Springfield, IL: Charles C. Thomas, 1987.

Zemlin, W. *Speech and Hearing Science*, Englewood Cliffs, NJ: Prentice-Hall, 1981.

ALANNA MCDONOUGH has a B.A. in psychology and linguistics and a M. Sc. in Communication Disorders. She is a practicing Speech Language Pathologist at the Foothills Hospital in Calgary and has specialized in Voice Disorders for the past 10 years. Alanna is also a clinical lecturer with the Department of Speech Pathology and Audiology at the University of Alberta. She is chair of the Universities Coordinating Council which reviews applicants for the Speech and Hearing Association of Alberta.

ELIZABETH J. HUNT, M.A., is director of the Voice Centre in Toronto. Ms. Hunt has 16 years of experience as a speech/language pathologist in Canada, the USA, and Australia. She has conducted research, provided treatment and taught seminars on care and use of the voice. She was a voice and dialect coach at Harvard University and is currently a faculty member in the Department of Speech and Language Pathology at the University of Toronto. Elizabeth has been a guest on television and radio and written articles for newspapers and professional journals.

ANNETTE HENDRIX is Administrative Assistant in the Faculty of Education, University of Calgary. She adapted these diagrams for publication in this chapter. Her baby girl arrived in July, 1995! Thus, three new "moms" contributed to this chapter.

Chapter 5
Accessing Trauma Through the Voice
Marcia J. Epstein

Let me begin by explaining what is intended here, which is the empowering of vocal sound as a healing modality. My company title, *Musica Humana*, is taken from a medieval treatise that refers to music as the science of proportion – including the proportions of the human body and of human society. Proportions internal and external, balances, symmetries, relationships, functions, harmonies: all are present in the body and the community. The medieval theorists of music knew and understood these relationships, and knew also that their art was equally a science. What they knew, we are now learning to discover all over again. Sound soothes, exhilarates, motivates, inspires, teaches and heals. The first musical instrument known to humanity was the voice, and we are rediscovering its wisdom.

I have been practicing Voice Therapy for approximately eighteen years now. It is useful to say so because the field doesn't officially exist yet, although there are already about two dozen expert practitioners on the North American continent alone. Very much alone until recently, in fact, since all of us call it something different, and we're just starting to network seriously. Voice Therapy is not the same as voice teaching, nor is it Music Therapy or Speech Therapy. Voice Therapy is equally an application of techniques and methods for correcting dysfunction in the voice, a belief in the efficacy of the voice as a diagnostic indicator for suppressed or unrecognized emotional states, and a recognition that vocal sound is therapeutic, both physically and emotionally. What we, its practitioners, are finding is that work on the voice is work on the *person*. It is fast and direct and no holds barred. It can speed up the process of traditional "talk" therapy and ground it in the body so that theory becomes practice, as gently and reasonably as taking a breath.

In fact, breath is crucial. So take a moment to be aware of yours – is it steady? Does it seem to reach all the way to your pelvic region; do your ribs flow around it smoothly; is it *welcome*? Important questions, because the holding of traumatic memories within the body/mind begins with holding the breath. It's what babies do when they're frightened, what adults do when they're tense and overworked and stressed out. If it becomes habitual, the voice may be constricted in tone, sounding tense or breathy or squeaky or harsh. Unlocking the voice begins with awareness of the breath: as the voice relaxes and expands, so does the body.

Voice Therapy involves breathing exercises, vocalizations and simple movements that are easily practiced in the client's home once the patterns become familiar through repetition. A few sample exercises are given at the end of this chapter and in the section on dysfunctional speech categories. Others may involve the use of arm and head movements, of walking in rhythm, of singing or humming a particular pattern of notes, of enunciating particular syllables repeatedly at varying speeds, or of measured breathing (e.g., inhale to a count of four beats, hold for four, exhale for four). A part of the effect of Voice Therapy comes from homework that accustoms the client to repatterning the breath and to listening for particular qualities of sound.

Listening, too, is crucial. North American culture is extremely visual, and most of our conditioning involves blocking out unwelcome sounds in an urban environment. At a 1993 conference held in Canada on the newly founded science of Acoustic Ecology, the study of sound in environments ranging from nature to urban culture, the trend in Western society toward increasing emphasis on vision was discussed in a cautionary context:

> *There is a final warning to be sounded about the ubiquity of the North American urban technologized soundscape. Paradoxically, it is increasingly visual. Music videos are a case in point: the listener is no longer trusted to envision a personal flow of images,*

and certainly not to let the music go by unvisualized. A current AT&T commercial, heralding the development of improved telephone reception, announces "Soon you will hear it" and the visual track flashes to a still picture of a human eye. In a culture dominated by visual media from print to video, what is seen is validated. It is no accident that in English speaking cultures, "hearsay" is a synonym for untruth. What, then, are we moving toward?" (Epstein, 1993).

The process of listening consciously is one that most of us are never taught unless we are judged at an early age to have talent in music. Even the training of musicians is often specifically focused on the idioms of particular instruments. Pianists, for example, may learn harmony more thoroughly than violinists because they play harmonies (several "lines" of music at once) while violinists more often play melodies (one "tune" at a time). French horn players become accustomed to an entirely different set of acoustic factors than harpists, and each develops selective hearing to some degree. Singers become adept at perceiving when another singer is about to breathe, a detail that usually escapes listeners without vocal training. This ability is important in choral performances: when the sound should continue uninterrupted for long periods of time: the singers of each separate part anticipate each others' breathing patterns in order to avoid breaking the continuity by breathing at the same time. Like musicians we all hear what we are taught to notice, and we tend not to hear what is not given attention. This latter category often includes our own voices.

In Western culture, children may be told that they are good looking, but rarely does anyone mention their voices except to insist that they be lowered indoors. We grow up largely unaware of our unique personal sounds, which serve to express individual identity, emotional state and family relations as surely as our visible traits and mannerisms. Our voiceprints, the visible charting of the wave forms and frequencies produced by our voices, are as individual as our fingerprints. The voice is a reflection of the myriad quirks and traits that make up a human being: genetic heritage, body structure, facial structure and musculature, early environment, temperament, vitality, emotional conditions, attitudes, stress levels. Even comfort zones, the individual's sense of ease and familiarity with a place or situation, are reflected in the voice, which may constrict or become hesitant in unfamiliar or nonsupportive surroundings.

The individual's relationship with his/her voice is often neglected unless some extreme condition – talent, desire or malfunction – brings it into full awareness. When that happens, an unexplored dimension of human nature may be revealed. In some cases, the voice and/or the breathing pattern has been impaired or damaged as a consequence of trauma experienced early in life. Trauma to the breath may result from chronic respiratory illnesses such as asthma, from physical damage to the lungs, trachea or face, or from frequent holding of the breath as a response to fear or physical pain. Impaired breathing patterns may manifest as constriction, shortness of breath, irregular or spasmodic breathing, or chronic breath holding. Trauma to the voice may be caused by injury to the larynx, throat or mouth, by chronic constriction due to fear, or by constant misuse of the voice related to unexpressed emotions: a "lump in the throat" sensation, for example, can become habitual if it is caused by longstanding grief or sorrow that has not been brought to awareness. The tension caused by a consistent habit of misuse can lead to the holding of a dysfunctional pattern, even in the absence of physical damage.

Dysfunctional patterns of breathing and vocalizing must be examined to discover causes. If the cause is purely physical, as when an accidental injury or physical abuse results in tissue damage, physical remedies or even surgery may be required. When the physical dysfunction results from chronic tension caused by a traumatic incident or by consistent emotional abuse or deprivation, the cure may be more complex. It often involves an emotional process of recalling memories about the traumatic situation, usually through some form of psychological counselling, combined with physical, mental and sometimes spiritual exercises designed to build and strengthen functional patterns of breathing and speaking to replace the dysfunctional ones. This latter process is the role of the Voice Therapist: to diagnose the relation of the dysfunction to previous trauma when that is indeed the cause, and to retrain the client's responses through the establishment of functional habits arrived at by repetition of exercises specific to the symptoms exhibited by the client. Such symptoms may include excessive harshness or breathiness in the voice, poor enunciation, inaudibility and/or visible constriction of the mouth and throat muscles.

It is important to remember that not all vocal dysfunction is caused by trauma – some of the many other possible causes are discussed in this chapter, as well. The exact category of trauma is also significant to the diagnosis. A car accident that injures the throat is traumatic, but it will not often cause chronic fear-related dysfunction. Once the physical damage is healed, the dysfunction usually fades. Illnesses in adulthood do not usually produce chronic dysfunction either. A severe respiratory illness in childhood, however, may do so. Constant physical and emotional abuse at any age may also relate to vocal dysfunction, though this does not by any means suggest that everyone with a vocal dysfunction has experienced abuse. My point here is not that trauma may be a cause of dysfunction – that much is obvious – but rather that treatment of the vocal dysfunction is an effective form of adjunct therapy for healing the longstanding physical and emotional results of trauma. Voice Therapy can enhance and speed the effects of both psychological and physiological modes of healing, and it needs to be regarded as one dimension of a multifaceted wholistic healing paradigm.

The process of coming to awareness of the causes for trauma-related dysfunction of the voice may uncover memories that are otherwise inaccessible, and help to resolve them. This is exactly what has happened for two of my clients, whose stories are presented here. The names of the two clients, "Barbara" and "Sarah," are pseudonyms designed to protect the privacy of both individuals. A few details not directly relevant to the case histories have been changed as well.

Case 1: "Barbara"

Barbara is a 43-year-old woman who began Voice Therapy because she was in her final stage of study for a Protestant ministry, and wanted to improve her public speaking skills.

She felt that her voice, which was clear and soft, needed more variety of expression for preaching and ceremonial tasks. Although she felt a deep sense of inspiration, Barbara suspected that neither her voice nor her public presence was conveying what she felt. At our first session, I noticed that her mouth and other facial muscles hardly moved, and that she was uncomfortable with walking while reading aloud, an exercise that often helps to "loosen" the voice by distracting the client from habitual physical tensions. This tendency toward immobility became more noticeable during the next session, and when I brought it to Barbara's attention she agreed that it was a longstanding habit of hers to move as little as possible. She also mentioned that she had some anxiety before coming to each session, because it felt "strange to make noise at all." Shortly after a third session, she phoned me to say that she had been thinking about possible reasons for the immobility and the anxiety, and had realized that they might pertain to the circumstances of her birth and early childhood.

Barbara was born in 1952 in a remote Czechoslovakian village, to a young mother who had been malnourished in her teens during World War II. The pregnancy strained her heart, and a doctor was present at the home birth. The baby, her first, was born after a six and a half month gestation and 72 hours of labor: a breech birth that produced an infant presumed stillborn. While the doctor and attendants worked to save the mother, the baby was wrapped up and set aside for "at least half an hour" until someone noticed her mouth moving slightly and realized she was alive. At that point, she was put into a basket with hot water bottles and fed with an eyedropper. Because of her prematurity, the baby's ears were covered with sheathing membranes and her skull elongated, a situation which did not normalize until she was some two and a half months old. Her lungs, too, were incompletely developed and she was unable to make noise. Kept swaddled the whole time, she was "remarkably static," and was discovered to have a malformed hip where dislocation had occurred during the birth.

When Barbara was nine months old, her mother left with her for Canada to join her husband, who had emigrated before the birth. Barbara was promptly put into a Canadian hospital and kept in a body cast from the chest down to correct the malformed hip. She remained in the cast until she was 18 months old, and was not able to walk unaided until she was three. Barbara states that she did not have any conscious memory of this stage of her life until 1985, when she experienced a sensation of "paralysis from the waist down" one night. Her husband was able to help her through the incident, and it did not recur. At this point, Barbara began to suspect that the circumstances of her birth might have been retained in some sort of "body memory" that affected her physical health long after the cast had been removed.

The concept of body memory is well established in several fields of alternative healing, and is now being researched and recognized in the medical paradigm of health. Among others, the works of Deepak Chopra (1991) and Larry Dossey (1991, 1982) – both medical doctors with an interest in alternative healing modes – translate the intricacy of medical models to the general public and explain the phenomena involved with self-healing. In one of several books on issues pertaining to health and healing, Dossey introduces the complexity of mind-body interaction as a philosophical problem:

> *The interaction of mind and matter and the way in which meaning affects the body involve the socalled mind-body problem, one of the most difficult questions in the history of Western philosophy. How can a thought, which seems and 'feels' nonphysical, alter cells, tissues, and organs, which seem overwhelmingly physical? How can such dissimilar things affect each other? It has never been clear to most persons who have thought deeply about this question how the actual interaction between atoms and thought takes place. When the mind affects the body it is as though some sort of magic has transpired, permitting material stuff somehow to be quickened by the mind. (Dossey, 1991, p. 20)*

The connection between mind and body remains mysterious. How does the chemistry of the human body alter at the instigation of an emotion, or even a memory of an emotion? How do we remember how to walk from one moment to the next? Why does an adult retain the physical responses appropriate to an experience from childhood, when that experience is not consciously remembered?

Let us begin the explication of body memory with a particularly vivid example. Chopra describes the "quantum mechanical body," which functions on physical and metaphysical levels simultaneously: "Here [in the "quantum" body] is where the trick of turning mind into matter is actually being managed. If you are frightened by meeting a snake in the woods, your heart starts to pound, your throat becomes dry, and your knees turn to rubber. By the time you jump back in fear, a split second transformation has taken place inside you. Your mental impulse – totally abstract and non-material – has manifested itself physically as molecules of adrenaline, which are concrete and totally material." (Chopra, 1991, p. 108)

Extending Chopra's scenario, we might envision returning to the spot where the snake was encountered, recognizing the location even though the snake is absent, and feeling a faint recurrence of the same phenomenon: a brief moment of pounding heart, dry throat and weak knees. This time, it is not the threat of danger itself but a recollection of an earlier threat that produces the mind to body signal, the abstraction manifested in the concrete world of scientific certainties.

Body memory has undoubtedly been known for centuries by musicians and athletes, who rely on constant practice to train their muscles to produce subtle responses instantly and automatically. When a musician learns a piece of music, the hands "remember" it even if years elapse between performances. Any habitual action is remembered by the body in the same way, particularly if it is started young. A lack of action, a state of immobility, can also be held and recalled as a pattern, and this appears to be one explanation for Barbara's experience. The combination of injury and enforced immobility produced in her two aspects of an experience of trauma that was "held" in her posture, mannerisms and speech into adulthood. The third, and perhaps definitive, aspect was prolonged lack of contact with her parents during a critical time for bonding with them.

Since the visitation rules during the time of her hospitalization were extremely restrictive, Barbara did not see her mother more than two hours per week while she was in the body cast, and hardly saw her father at all. He stopped visiting, she says, because he didn't think she remembered him. Later he left the family, and eventually stopped contacting them. Barbara knew very little about him until 1993, when his brother contacted her from Berlin and filled in several details of the family history, one of which was the fact that on her father's side, Barbara was descended from generations of Protestant clergy and church musicians. Upon learning this history, she felt that her call to enter the clergy became even stronger, and that she wanted to be able to express her inspiration more fully. This decision led her to a desire to improve her speaking, and to a reconnection of the fragments of memory from her early childhood. She began to interview members of her mother's family about the incidents of her birth. The beginning of Voice Therapy sessions led her to further connect the memories and family stories with her present situation.

Once I became acquainted with Barbara's account of her early history, I prescribed some simple physical exercises to explore and overcome her sense of physical restriction. These included crawling on hands and knees to simulate the experience of a baby learning motor coordination: because of her injury and hospitalization, she had not experienced this stage of movement at the critical age. Barbara reported that at first the movements were "jerky and awkward. They took all my physical and emotional energy – I could sustain them for only about five minutes at a time. I had to be alone in the house to do them at all. Then I began to grunt with the effort – involuntary sounds – and then I started to make noises for excitement and release, only while moving." The "whoops, hollers and laughs" produced by the physical exercises were the first sign that Barbara's childhood was being healed and repatterned. The process of relearning the mind-body connection released a level of spontaneity that had not been part of her previous experience. She is now exploring the influence of her early childhood more fully and learning to work with her breathing patterns consciously in order to develop her voice and public presence. Exercises that she now practices, designed for her particular focus, include "Breathing the Holy

Spirit" and "Waterfall Sounds." (See the end of this chapter for instructions.)

Barbara's case presents an example of how the voice is connected to somatic responses and restrictions, and how its development corresponds with the changing of conditioned patterns. The release of sound accompanies the release of muscular response patterns, and can be used as a barometer to gauge progress in self-healing. A second example of trauma, the case of Sarah, illustrates the effects on the voice of physical and sexual abuse in childhood.

Case 2: "Sarah"

Sarah is a 32-year-old woman who began Voice Therapy in order to expand the range of her speaking voice, which was extremely high pitched and breathy, giving her a hesitant and childish sound. We began working with a series of vocalizations that were designed to relax the laryngeal muscles and increase breath control. These included exercises to increase the volume and range of the voice, as well as heightened speech, in which the client learns to read aloud in inflected patterns resembling chants – part speech, part song and very emphatic. Sarah made progress with the exercises, increasing her awareness of the variety of sounds available to her, but her voice remained tense.

During the third of her Voice Therapy sessions, Sarah informed me that she was a survivor of childhood incest, and that she had completed a course of psychological counselling that enabled her to recognize and process the issues involved. There were, however, still some unexplained symptoms and reactions that troubled her, and she suspected that the constriction of her voice was related to the abuse she had experienced. For this reason, she was combining the voice development work with cranial-sacral therapy, a form of bodywork that identifies and enhances the subtle flows of energy along the spine with techniques related to therapeutic touch, polarity and acupressure massage. It is a very subtle and gentle process that produces marked changes in posture, gait and musculature, freeing the body of habitual tensions.

Sarah's early home life had been a casebook nightmare. Her father, who was hospitalized repeatedly for severe bipolar disorder (formerly known as manic-depressive disorder), was physically and sexually abusive to Sarah and her younger brother when he was left alone with them. In Sarah's case the abuse included damage to the muscles of her throat by sexual molestation, as well as an incident of being held underwater in the bathtub. Threatened with death if they told anyone, the children did not mention the abuse even to each other until many years later, and their mother claimed to have no knowledge of it. Sarah's father was now forbidden by court order to approach her.

Among Sarah's remaining symptoms was an occasional tendency to lose her voice completely while speaking on the phone. She reported, upon arrival for her fifth session with me, that this had happened to her earlier that day. She had caught a glimpse of her father in a downtown crowd, and phoned her husband, but was unable to speak. She described her throat as "frozen." Although she assured me that there was no actual danger to her at this time, she was visibly agitated. We began the session with a guided meditation in which I encouraged Sarah to envision a safe and comforting environment, and then to ask herself whether there was a story her throat wanted to tell her: such personification of body parts and systems is standard practice in guided imagery work, because it allows the client to set up a dialogue in which previously unacknowledged memories can be conveyed in a nonthreatening manner. During the process, the client is given gentle encouragement to verbalize any information that feels appropriate, but is not required to do so. The dialogue may remain internal if that is perceived as the more safe route. The session always ends with the facilitator guiding the client back to safety and then into waking consciousness. To this standard practice of visualization and dialogue, I add instructions to the client to feel free to express any abstracts sounds, noises or songs that occur during the process. Such preverbal vocalizations can be important clues to the client's emotional state and physical condition, as well as an effective mechanism for the release of stored tensions. Preverbal sounds – groans, chortles, yips, yells, hums, babbling, laughter and many other sounds along the entire emotional spectrum – are the language of human infancy. They can serve to put the adult client in touch with early childhood emotions and experiences, and to release the childlike qualities of spontaneity and play. They can also provide a safe process for recalling traumatic incidents and releasing the fear associated with them.

The memory held in Sarah's throat emerged in part during the guided meditation, and in part afterward. She had re-experienced a memory, from the age of twelve, of attempting to phone the police for help when her father threatened her. Finding her with phone in hand, he had attempted to strangle her, silencing her voice. It was this "muscle memory," unconscious until the guided imagery session, that had been constricting her voice on the telephone ever since. Once the memory was recognized, the symptom stopped occurring.

Sarah has since reported that the voice work has begun to "thaw what was frozen" in her throat, and made her aware of the reasons for her vocal constrictions. It has also increased in her a desire to overcome her vocal limitations. She reported to me that at the end of the guided meditation, during the resurfacing phase, she interpreted my instruction to "reassure the throat muscles" by telling them that the danger was gone, and they did not have to protect her by tensing. They then "asked," "What do we do now?" Her intuition replied to them: "Create a beautiful and joyous voice." She is now well on the way to doing so.

Applications of Voice Therapy Outside the Context of Trauma

Many of the approaches applicable to dealing with trauma are also appropriate for the voice that is simply fatigued, constricted, harsh or weak. Not every vocal problem can be traced to a traumatic situation; many are the result of improper breathing or speaking techniques, or of modelling the voice in childhood on a parent whose speech was dysfunctional. Many people model their voices unconsciously in childhood on the voice of the same sex parent, imitating pitch, volume, inflections, accent and mannerisms as accurately as a recording. Heredity, too, plays a part: the structure of the child's facial bones and the shape of the larynx and sinuses may duplicate those of a parent, and contribute to particular tonal characteristics in the voice. When a voice is dysfunctional, some basic corrections may improve it. These include attention to breathing, to relaxation of muscle tensions in the face, jaw, neck, shoulders, upper back and abdomen, and to inflection. While corrections of dysfunctional speech are best done on an individual basis, with the coach or therapist devoting time to the specific needs of each client, some general principles can be suggested so that minor difficulties may be overcome in the absence of a trained specialist.

In my work with the Teaching Development Office at the University of Calgary, I have had many opportunities to correct dysfunctional speech patterns in people who make a living with their voices, as university instructors. A brief and partial survey of common speech problems, gathered from their ranks, may serve here to suggest some effective approaches to specific difficulties. The problems may be categorized in three ways: dysfunctions of volume, tone, inflection and speed.

Dysfunctions of Volume.

1. Weak or excessively soft speech.

The emotional cause is generally shyness, or fear of public speaking. Usually the physical problem is lack of air: the breath is shallow or held while speaking. Correction may be as simple as practicing the Basic Breathing Lesson (see Sample Exercises) in order to develop the habit of abdominal breathing. "Chest breathers," who puff their chests and heave their shoulders upward when asked to take a deep breath, are not breathing correctly and often develop respiratory problems as well as weaknesses in speech. Abdominal breathing is natural to all animals, including humans. For a model of how to breathe well, watch a dog or a human infant in the process. The "ha!" exercise (see "Excessive Breathiness" on the following page) is also useful.

2. Harsh or excessively loud speech.

The emotional cause may be unexpressed anger, frustration or resentment. The physical problem is constriction of the muscles of the throat and jaw, and holding the breath while shouting from the throat. If the problem persists, it may lead to vocal nodes – tiny lumps on the vocal cords that must be removed by surgery. Correction may be accomplished by a combination of Basic (abdominal) Breathing exercises and practicing a "breathy" tone to modify the harshness. "Waterfall Sounds" (see Sample Exercises) that involve sighing or whooshing noises can be used to induce breathiness.

Dysfunctions of Tone

1. Nasality

A "nasal" voice is usually caused by tension in the muscles of the mouth and jaw. Massaging the muscles surrounding the mouth, and along the lower jaw to the ears, may be helpful. Practice in "dropping the jaw" is also important: let the mouth hang halfway open in a relaxed position, and concentrate on keeping it relaxed while speaking. A habit of tensing the corners of the mouth in a habitual grimace is common with nasal voices, and can be overcome with attention to gentle vertical motions of the jaw and relaxation of the mouth.

2. Excessive breathiness

A "breathy" voice is one that does not engage the vocal cords in full vibration. It may also be associated with shallow breathing (see previous section on "Weak or excessively soft speech"). Correction may involve abdominal breathing (see "Basic Breathing Lesson" in Sample Exercises) and practicing the connection between breath and voice projection by shouting a series of "ha!" and "ho!" sounds, pulsing the diaphragm slightly inward with each syllable.

3. "Machine gun" speech

"Machine gun" speech is excessively abrupt, with each word or syllable overenunciated and unconnected to the flow of the syntax. Correction may involve the "Waterfall Sounds" exercise (see Sample Exercises) and relaxation of the mouth and jaw muscles with massage and slackening exercises (for an example, see "Nasality"). Jaw movement while speaking should be minimized.

4. *"Slack jaw" speech*

"Slack jaw" speech is mumbled and underenunciated. The jaw muscles need to be activated by smiling and employing the mouth muscles consciously while reading aloud. "Basic Breathing" (see Sample Exercises) is also essential.

Dysfunctions of Inflection

1. *Monotone*

Monotone is the habit of speaking on one pitch. It may be associated with nasality or "machine gun" speech, and often results from tension in the jaw. As with both conditions cited above, massage and slackening exercises can help. It is also associated with holding the breath while speaking. Both "Basic Breathing" and "Waterfall Sounds" (see Sample Exercises) are useful, followed by exercises that involve reading aloud with exaggerated pitch variation.

2. *Excessively high pitch*

Associated with overuse of the arytenoid (upper laryngeal) muscles. "Waterfall Sounds" (see Sample Exercises) and reading aloud with exaggerated pitch variation can be helpful as correctives. Singing lessons are extremely helpful.

3. *Excessively low pitch*

Associated with overuse of the cryco-thyroid (lower laryngeal) muscles. As with high pitch, "Waterfall Sounds" (see Sample Exercises) and reading aloud with exaggerated pitch variation can be helpful as correctives. Singing lessons are extremely helpful.

Dysfunctions of Speed

1. *Excessively fast speech*

May be associated with strong enthusiasm, or with excessive anxiety. Awareness of the breath and of enunciation is crucial. Reading aloud with a metronome, set to approximately 60, is helpful to produce a sense of measured rhythm. Walking slowly with relaxed arms and legs, swinging the arms in time to the metronome, is also useful.

2. Excessively slow speech

May be associated with "slack jaw" speech (see above), and with fear of public speaking. "Basic Breathing" (see Sample Exercises) is essential. Reading the same passage aloud several times, increasing speed with each repetition, is helpful (change passages occasionally to avoid boredom). Gradually change from reading to spontaneous improvised speech.

Conclusions and Cautions

It is important to point out here that developing the voice is not an isolated activity separate from development of motor skills, breathing patterns, sensory awareness, memory, emotional expression and personality. It is not a "cure" for trauma-related conditions, but rather an effective adjunct therapy to be used in conjunction with psychotherapy or psychological counselling, and/or with bodywork. The voice itself is intimately connected to both physical and emotional states, and its malfunctions are symptomatic of malfunctions elsewhere in the human system. For that reason, it is important for anyone using vocalization as a therapeutic mode to have expert training in vocal technique, so that the difference between free and constricted sound, as well as the range of the human vocal spectrum, can be recognized. If the practitioner is not clinically trained as well, it is advisable to form an alliance with certified counsellors and/or bodyworkers for client referrals. In working with the development or correction of the voice, personal issues may arise that are beyond the expertise of the voice teacher or speech therapist, and technical problems may manifest that are beyond the expertise of the psychologist or bodyworker. A team approach is most effective when evidence of trauma presents itself in a client. The process of recognizing and describing the source of the trauma, be it as minor as a childhood anxiety or as major as a history of abuse, is bound to affect the "voice" in both the physical and psychological senses of the term. Practitioners who work with the physical voice and counsellors who work with the emotional voice would do well to learn from each others' wisdom, and to collaborate. What will be born from their association is a new science.

At this, the onset of the twenty-first century, we are beginning to recognize the true complexity of health and health care. It is not just a matter of treating the body in isolation from the mind, nor of alleviating symptoms without fully comprehending and addressing their causes. There is room on the same continuum for the expertise of physicians, nurses, counsellors, bodyworkers and arts based alternative practitioners such as music, voice and dance therapists. What is required of the client is a deep and genuine curiosity about how (s)he has evolved as a person, and how that process of growth can be continued to encompass previously unknown experiences and abilities. What is required of the practitioner is dedication, expert training, a keen eye for observing, a sensitive ear for listening, and the ability to follow intuition wherever it leads. With these elements, true healing can be accomplished.

Sample Exercises for Expanding Awareness of the Breath and the Voice

1. Basic Breathing Lesson – **for breathing with the full capacity of the lungs**

- Stand with your feet flat on the floor or ground, slightly apart. Relax your shoulders and flex your knees slightly.

- Place one hand on your chest, the other on your abdominal muscles (just below the waist). Do not press, just place the hands to rest lightly on your body: they will serve to draw your awareness to the elements of the breathing process.

- Let out all your breath through slightly pursed lips. Your abdomen should contract slightly.

- Inhale slowly by ballooning the abdominal muscles gently outward and downward against your hand, so that you can feel the air coming in. The breath will move to the midsection, and finally expand your chest very slightly. Do not puff out the chest, just let it fill gently with air. Do not move your shoulders at all, except to relax them.

- Exhale by gently contracting the abdominal muscles toward your spine.

- Repeat the process several times. If you become dizzy, rest for awhile, then try again.

This is the way we are designed to breathe: not with the chest and shoulders in a state of tension, but with the entire body. Breathe this way all the time.

2. Breathing the Holy Spirit – for experiencing inspiration.

- Stand with your feet bare, about shoulder width apart, hands relaxed at sides, eyes closed.

- Breathe gently and deeply, through the nose; expanding the abdominal muscles first, then the chest. Notice the breath filling your lungs and gently rocking your body.

- Imagine that there is an angel standing behind you, breathing into a point at the base of your skull, just where it meets your spine, breathing comfort and love into you. Envision the breath as golden white light which fills your body with a sense of well-being and glowing health.

- Ask the angel to bless your breath and your health.

- To conclude the exercise, concentrate on your feet. Move your feet and hands gently, then open your eyes. For best effect, write about what you envisioned and felt so that you can recall it later. Practice this exercise when you want inspiration (e.g., for beginning a project, or facing a test) or comfort.

3. Waterfall Sounds – for releasing inhibitions about the use of the voice.

- Stand with your feet approximately shoulder width apart, hands relaxed at sides, eyes closed (they may be opened, if you prefer, once you become accustomed to the exercise), knees slightly flexed.

- Imagine that your breath is circling up the back of your spine from the floor or ground under your feet as you inhale, reaching the top of your head, then cascading like a waterfall down the front of your body to your feet. Release the "waterfall" exhalation without controlling it – just let it out. Let your head and shoulders bend slightly forward with each exhalation.

- Add sound to the exhalation, moving from high to low. It can be a whoosh, a sigh, a groan, an "ah" or other open vowel sound, or any other relaxed sound that occurs to you. You may use the same sound with each exhale, or change sounds, as you please. Let the sound get a little bit louder with each exhalation.

- To conclude the exercise, resume normal posture and breath gradually.

Recommended Readings:

Campbell, D. *Music and Miracles*. Wheaton, IL: Quest Books, 1992.

Campbell, D. *The Roar of Silence*. Wheaton, IL: Quest Books, 1989.

Chopra, D. *Perfect Health*. New York: Crown Publishing, 1991.

Dossey, L. *Meaning and Medicine*. New York: Bantam Books, 1991.

Dossey, L. *Space, Time, and Medicine*. Boston: Shambhala Publications, 1982.

Epstein, M. J. *ReSounding the BodyMind: Explorations in Metaphysiology*. (Work in Progress, 1995.)

Epstein, M. J. "SOUND BARRIERS: Reverberations on Prehistory, Technology, and Culture", in *"The Tuning of the World": Proceedings of the First International Conference on Acoustic Ecology* (1993). Banff, AB: The Banff Centre, 1994. (available on audiotape only).

Zi, N. *The Art of Breathing*. New York: Bantam Books, 1986.

And Special Thanks to extraordinary voice teachers:
Ken Nielsen and Persis Ensor.

MARCIA JENNETH EPSTEIN, Ph.D., is a cultural historian, musician and composer. In her academic life, she teaches for the Faculty of General Studies at the University of Calgary, in a program of interdisciplinary courses that trace the thematic paradigms in Western culture. At present, research interests include Acoustic Ecology, Music Therapy and alternatives modes of healing with voice and sound. As a performer, she is a singer trained in the classical traditions of both the West and of Northern India, and a voice coach with eighteen years of experience in helping people to overcome fears and dysfunctions related to the use of the voice for singing and speaking. Her clientèle includes educators, actors and singers, as well as people who have always wanted to sing and were told not to.

Chapter 6
Your Story

Your voice is an unique characteristic, reflecting your life experiences just as surely as does your fingerprint or foot print. Therefore, this chapter is yours: give "voice" to your ideas about how you might care for your teaching or coaching voice. Perhaps the following suggestions, offered by teachers who took an In-Service course on voice, will be useful. Use them as a workbook for analyzing your voice and planning for the care of your voice.

Complete the sentences:

**When I think about my voice, I am mainly con-
cerned with . . .**

**When I think about my voice, I am mainly pleased
with . . .**

What qualities does my voice express now?

What qualities would I like it to express?

What are my goals with regard to caring for my voice?

With whose story in the previous chapters did I most identify? Why?

What strategies might I use to maintain or develop strengths?

What strategies might I use to reduce pathologies?

How would I recognize improvement in my voice?

Notes

Notes

Notes

Notes

Notes

Notes